T0034409

ADHD Girls to Women

of related interest

Understanding ADHD in Girls and Women
Edited by Joanne Steer
Foreword by Andrea Bilbow OBE
ISBN 978 1 78775 400 3
eISBN 978 1 78775 401 0

The Teenage Girl's Guide to Living Well with ADHD
Improve your Self-Esteem, Self-Care and Self Knowledge
Sonia Ali
ISBN 978 1 78775 768 4
eISBN 978 1 78775 769 1

ADHD an A–Z
Figuring it Out Step by Step
Leanne Maskell
ISBN 978 1 83997 385 7
eISBN 978 1 83997 386 4

ADHD
Girls to Women

Getting on the Radar

Lotta Borg Skoglund

Forewords by Professor Susan Young and
Ann-Kristin Sandberg

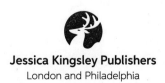

Jessica Kingsley Publishers
London and Philadelphia

First published in Great Britain in 2024 by Jessica Kingsley Publishers
An imprint of John Murray Press

1

Copyright © Lotta Borg Skoglund 2024
Translation copyright © Alison Wheather 2024
Forewords copyright © Professor Susan Young and Ann-Kristin Sandberg 2024

The right of Lotta Borg Skoglund to be identified as the Author of the Work has been
asserted by them in accordance with the Copyright, Designs and Patents Act 1988.

All rights reserved. No part of this publication may be reproduced, stored
in a retrieval system, or transmitted, in any form or by any means without
the prior written permission of the publisher, nor be otherwise circulated
in any form of binding or cover other than that in which it is published and
without a similar condition being imposed on the subsequent purchaser.

Content warning: This book mentions eating disorders.

A CIP catalogue record for this title is available from the
British Library and the Library of Congress

ISBN 978 1 80501 054 8
eISBN 978 1 80501 055 5

Printed and bound in Great Britain by TJ Books Ltd

Jessica Kingsley Publishers' policy is to use papers that are natural,
renewable and recyclable products and made from wood grown in
sustainable forests. The logging and manufacturing processes are expected
to conform to the environmental regulations of the country of origin.

Jessica Kingsley Publishers
Carmelite House
50 Victoria Embankment
London EC4Y 0DZ

www.jkp.com

John Murray Press
Part of Hodder & Stoughton Ltd
An Hachette Company

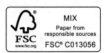

MIX
Paper from
responsible sources
FSC
www.fsc.org   FSC® C013056

I've lived my entire life with the knowledge that I'm not like everyone else. Still, I've always believed in what others tell me – that my belief that my experiences, my problems, and my emotional register are different is all in my head.

I've tried, given up, and started again so many times, always with the feeling that I can achieve it as long as I try hard enough. To be normal. Everyone else manages it, right? I've never understood why I'm so stupid and lazy. Why don't I just do things properly straight off or learn from my mistakes? But I'm not lazy. I don't know anyone who's struggled as hard as I have.

It wasn't until I was diagnosed and got the right treatment that I realized that you can be tired without being sad. That you can be sad without being hungry, and that it's perfectly safe to be bored sometimes.

Now I know that I'm not stupid, not lazy, and not useless. My diagnosis has given me a deep and sincere love for myself and a great feeling of humility towards life. Not only can I take better care of myself, but I can also be a better mum, friend, partner, and colleague.

It's quite strange. The more you take care of yourself, the more energy you have for other things. It's not as if all the clouds have dispersed and I'm a new person now that I've had my diagnosis. I'm still the same Lina, with bouts for emotional turmoil, and slumps of self-confidence that are easily triggered by stress and anxiety. The difference is that I'm no longer afraid and ashamed of myself.

I know it's all passing storms and I'm constantly working on the courage to sit still in the boat when it's windy – and to grab the oars and row when it's still. But it's so very much easier to be in charge and work with yourself when you understand how you operate, that it's a question of biology and not choice. My diagnosis has created a win-win-win-win situation – for me, for my family, for my colleagues, and for society in general. I can now take responsibility of my own part in this, take better care of myself, and live a rich, healthy, and dignified life.

Lotta, 48

Contents

Foreword by Professor Susan Young

My journey leading to a career in clinical psychology, specializing in ADHD and Autism, commenced in 1993 when I did my PhD at the Institute of Psychiatry, Psychology and Neuroscience (King's College London). My PhD was an eight-year follow-up community study of 7-year-old girls who had been previously identified as having ADHD symptoms, conduct problems or neither. The aim was to investigate the long-term outcome of ADHD in girls (in those days referred to as 'hyperactive girls'). I visited and interviewed them all in their homes when they were 15–16 years old. I was pregnant at the time, and I recall completing the interviews in the nick of time – the last one being within my due date window!

I remember the girls well. One was pregnant, she didn't have her own bedroom and she slept in bed with her mother. Several of the girls talked to me about suicidal ideations, attempts and self-harming behaviours; one disclosed to me that she had impulsively taken a substantial amount of paracetamol in an attempt to take her life the day before. Many of the girls talked about emotional dysregulation; some had violent outbursts and I recall one girl pulling out a knife she had secreted under her chair 'just in case'. They were often in trouble at school, getting detentions and many of them truanted. Academically they didn't do well; two of the girls had left school without taking exams so they had no qualifications. One of them got a job in retail sales but was fired days later. Peer relationships were damaged; they described feeling socially isolated. Nearly all of them lacked a social network of supportive friendships; they didn't have people to talk to about their problems or share their secrets with. Some had good relationships with their family but others did not. What was very clear was that they lacked functional coping strategies, so when they faced difficulties and troubles – as many teenagers do at this age – they were lost. They lived for the day and never thought of the future; they were leaves in the wind.

I've never forgotten those girls. Today, they would be around 45 years old and I have often wondered what became of them. This book gives me the answers – Lotta Skoglund achieves her aim to 'describe what it can be like to live with ADHD, as a female and in different stages of life'. We know, unfortunately, that for years girls and women with ADHD have fallen 'under the radar'. Because they are not 'boisterous boys' meeting stereotypical expectations of how ADHD presents, they are unidentified. They are the invisible group who struggle alone, often accumulating more and more distress, disappointment, frustration and despair as they move forward in life. Some people talk about ADHD to be their 'superpower'; few of them are women and this term simply undermines the effort it takes to manage their struggles and camouflage their difficulties. This book captures their journey. There are good times, there are bad times and there are tempests. Thinking back to those girls I interviewed all those years ago, I wonder whether any of them were diagnosed and treated and, if so, was their outcome better?

Peppered with heart-felt vignettes, that will resonate with many readers and in 'user friendly' language, this book provides a psychoeducational focus that demystifies ADHD and its diagnosis. Lotte describes what's going on in the ADHD brain, the interface with hormonal change and co-existing psychiatric conditions. She explains how ADHD impacts on individuals' expectations of themselves and those of others, and how it affects life satisfaction and personal wellbeing. She explains how it impacts on the different roles that we juggle across life domains – home, school, work, social, pregnancy, motherhood, partnerships, friendships, family. She considers how this changes over time (child, adolescence, mid-life and older). Lotte is not afraid to say it how it is. She addresses the difficulties head on; this will reassure the reader that they are not alone in feeling overwhelmed and unable to cope when things build up inside - that, feeling misunderstood and alone, some women turn to alcohol and drugs to get them through. Importantly Lotte turns to positive interventions, both professional and personal. A beacon of hope.

Every healthcare practitioner and allied professional working with girls and women with ADHD should read this book. Every girl and woman who has ADHD, or who believes they may have ADHD, should read it. It will give them a sense of validation, to know that there are people 'out there' who understand them and who 'get' them. It will inform their understanding of themselves, answering questions of 'how' and 'why'. It will guide them to think about 'what' in their future. It will help them to recognize that they do not have to be leaves in the wind.

Professor Susan Young, BSc, PhD, DClinPsy, CPsychol, CSci, AFBPS
www.psychology-services.uk.com

Foreword by Ann-Kristin Sandberg

When first hearing the term attention deficit hyperactivity disorder (ADHD), most people still think of a disruptive or mischievous boy. Boys tend to exhibit more externalizing behaviour that is heard and seen in a way that few will miss. Consequently, the difficulties and specific needs of girls and women easily get overlooked, as they often express themselves in other ways. ADHD in girls and women is often detected later than in boys, causing unnecessary suffering, with sometimes serious consequences. The reality behind these dire inequalities is what this book addresses and is why I read it with great curiosity.

Lotta Borg Skoglund fills a gap in our knowledge of what it's like to be a girl or a woman living with ADHD. In an exemplary fashion, she reaches beyond diagnostic criteria and symptom descriptions, although these matters are also discussed. One of the book's many strengths is the life stories that foster a genuine understanding of the challenges with which the women have wrestled during their lives. Awareness and recognition are valuable, especially for those seeking help and support.

In my experience, many people find it hard to believe that someone who seems to function so well on the surface could be struggling with an underlying chaos that makes it difficult to manage what others do so easily. Far too often, incapacity is interpreted as unwillingness. The individual seeking help risks not being taken seriously, which reinforces their feelings of being an outlier, a failure.

Lotta also addresses the popular debate on ADHD, which simplistically emphasizes different strengths that are claimed to accompany the diagnosis – qualities like creativity, courage, innovativeness, curiosity, and an ability to see what others do not. Some people even refer to ADHD as a superpower. The truth, however, is often quite different. In this book, we read about women who struggle to get through the day, never understanding why everything always becomes so much harder and more complicated for them.

In many situations, the behavioural expectations on girls and women are still unfairly high. This puts an enormous pressure on those with ADHD who already try exceedingly hard to be accepted. Not being able to accomplish what other people seem to do so easily gives rise to constant stress and sinking self-esteem. As girls enter adulthood, the expectations to hold down a job and a family can prove too much, and far too many young women end up on sick leave for depression or burnout. The way back from there is, unfortunately, often very long.

Disseminating facts and raising awareness in society about the difficulties of ADHD is an important part of improving the support of this severely underserved group. They need support to combat the negative consequences that ADHD often has on their health, academic and work life performances, personal relationships, and livelihoods.

Occasionally, I have heard healthcare professionals describe ADHD as 'lightweight psychiatry'. Naturally, there are considerable individual differences in severity and level of functional impairment, but what we need to bear in mind is that many people with ADHD live more demanding lives than others, regardless of what is seen from the outside. Data from various studies indicates a distinctly elevated risk – at the group level – of serious healthcare needs, sick leave, unemployment, divorce, shortened life expectancy, and suicide.

Of course, each person with ADHD has unique potential – but freeing it requires better conditions than those currently offered by society. Every individual with ADHD needs individualized and tailored support in school, decent healthcare without long waiting times, and a welcoming working environment with appropriate accommodations.

This book provides a thorough account of what is currently understood about the ADHD brain, the significance of sex and gender, what it's like to live with ADHD, and what kind of support and accommodations are recommended. It opens a window onto the tough reality that many women have to endure, but it also offers hope through testimonies of improved self-efficacy and effective therapies. The chances of feeling better and being able to cope with life are good – if you seek and receive support.

In closing, the book predicts what the future looks like for this group. Lotta shares the hopes of my organization – Attention – that we will eventually understand and respond better to girls and women with ADHD on the basis of the unique challenges that nature and our social structures impose on them. This book will therefore be an important tool in creating a less prejudiced and more accepting society in which individuals are allowed to be themselves without being pressured to conform to normative stereotypes.

I hope it gains wide circulation among women, their families, the professionals who meet them, and the rest of us who want to learn more about ADHD.

Ann-Kristin Sandberg
Department head of The Swedish National
Patient Association for ADHD, Attention

Struggling Uphill and Running Aground

I'm a general practitioner and psychiatrist specializing in ADHD, addiction, and other comorbidities particularly prevalent among children and adults with neurodevelopmental disorders. I'm also an associate professor of psychiatry at Uppsala University and Karolinska Institutet, and my research over the years has come to focus on gender aspects of neurodevelopmental disorders, addiction, emotional dysregulation, reproductive health, and sex hormones in ADHD. During my years as a doctor, I have met so many girls and women who have struggled heartbreakingly hard just to make the basic things in life work. Despite their intelligence or talents, white knuckles, and constant restarts, they tell me that they simply can't get their lives into gear. Regrettably, neither the scientific community nor healthcare services have shown any real interest in the unique challenges facing girls and women with ADHD, and frighteningly little is still understood about this large group of struggling and severely underserved people.

If this sounds all too relatable, this book is for you.

I intended to write a book outlining the research on the

uniqueness of ADHD in girls and women. I soon realized this wouldn't be a particularly thick book – more a leaflet, or at most, a booklet. After plumbing the depths of the literature pool on ADHD, I found that the women's end is dangerously shallow. Diving there is certainly not advisable! So, if the ADHD researchers (with some important exceptions, please note) have not thought it important enough to study the differences between females and males with ADHD, why do I, a psychiatrist and researcher specializing in ADHD, still insist that gender aspects must be addressed? Why do we need to discuss sex differences? Shouldn't we all be treated the same, regardless of sex, gender, or diagnosis? In a utopian world, it would be a given that we are offered medical and personal treatment on the basis of our individual characteristics. Unfortunately, that is not the case, yet. And whether we like it or not, there are important biological differences between men and women to consider.

But can support and treatment currently given for ADHD be considered fair and equal if it is based on the male norm? I don't think so. Furthermore, if we disregard how the bodies and brains of men and women are constructed, treating everyone the same will have consequences for those who need to adapt to the accepted norm. We overlook girls with ADHD because we're looking for symptoms that are common in boys. We lose girls and young women from effective treatment because most pharmacological studies on drugs and doses are done on boys and men.

ADHD is the same disorder in both sexes, but as we'll understand from the stories in this book, it can present in various different ways. Both biological differences and a society that persists in imposing different social and cultural expectations on girls and boys, women and men, contribute to this.

The personal stories and testimonies shared in this book are real, though often personal details have been changed to protect their identities. All the women and girls featured have consented to me sharing their stories and, in fact, many urged me to tell them in the hope that others may identify with their struggles.

They have much to teach us. They have all found ways through or around the difficulties their ADHD has brought them – clever strategies and ingenious, helpful solutions that they want to share with others.

This book does not offer a magic bullet fashioned from self-help handbooks. Nor is it a comprehensive or exhaustive overview of ADHD. Nonetheless, in light of my experience of the support and treatment recommended through evidence-based guidelines, these tips and tricks complement traditional healthcare treatments and offerings. My sincere wish is that by providing others with important tools such as self-efficacy, self-respect, and responsibility for oneself, individuals can gain inspiration and guidance, regardless of any diagnosis.

Recently, it seems there has been a lot more of a push from media for those struggling with mental health and parenting children with challenges to 'pull yourself together'. Not uncommonly, these oversimplified narratives tend to also revolve around ADHD and other 'letter combinations' and it sometimes seems as if 'everyone has to have some kind of combination of something nowadays'.

However, when I talk about ADHD, I don't mean children, teenagers, and adults who have suddenly hit rock bottom or who struggle sometimes when life is tough. On the contrary, these are more typically *entire lives* spent relentlessly struggling uphill and running aground, frequently without any firm diagnosis or with multiple diagnoses in different combinations. But often there is no one specific diagnosis that really seems to pinpoint the problem.

Indeed, in ADHD it is quite common that hours, weeks, or even years of misguided and costly therapy result in incorrect medications and flawed advice. This misinformed guidance is problematic for the individual who has never understood her 'gut instincts' or for whom there are hundreds of conflicting instincts to follow. When searching for answers without first obtaining an appropriate explanatory model, it's easy to act on misguided advice from the majority – that is, those without ADHD.

Many girls and women tell me that for as long as they can remember, they have lived in a state of constant doubt about themselves and their self-worth. A good many have known from an early age that 'something is not right' and that they are 'different somehow' but never found the right words for these nagging, shameful feelings. ADHD manifests differently from person to person. Therefore, many women fumble their way through life, easy prey to self-help cures or well-meaning but ignorant samaritans. Maybe they wonder why their inner motor never seems to stop, and how they should get all their parallel trains of thought under control. Or they ask why their engine won't start when they know they have important things to get done. Or why they start one thing, forget another, flounder over a third, and drop a fourth to the floor. Why is it so hard to remain in the moment and listen and why are their thoughts always wandering off somewhere else? Many feel banished, as if they can never fit in, and, ultimately, many will experience extreme and tormenting loneliness.

We now know, thanks to extensive research and long clinical experience, that ADHD is a neurodevelopmental, biological condition in which certain brain functions are significantly delayed in their maturity. We also actually know a great deal, but of course far from everything, about what underlies the problems ADHD causes. To then claim, in light of all this knowledge, that ADHD is a made-up diagnosis or an excuse for sloppy behaviour is a remarkable display of ignorance and arrogance.

We have enough research pointing out the costs to the individual and society if we do nothing. But it's also harmful to be given the wrong explanatory model and consequently the wrong treatment. In worst-case scenarios, certain pharmacological treatments or therapies will not only delay proper diagnosing but can aggravate the ADHD symptoms. Furthermore, repeated misguided psychological interventions can prove detrimental for the individual who will constantly fail to act on flawed advice that doesn't take the underlying ADHD into consideration.

So, how can it be that such a common and well-understood diagnosis is still so controversial and contentious? And how can it be that so many people live almost their entire lives before realizing that their ADHD has created a pattern of impediment and failure? There are probably as many reasons as there are people with ADHD. However, one important reason why we miss and misunderstand this diagnosis is that ADHD can present itself so differently in different people. Another is that ADHD can be displayed so differently at various periods of the same person's life. A third is that it becomes so difficult for both the person with the diagnosis and others around her to comprehend that what might work one day will not work the next.

Today, we recognize ADHD as a dimensional or continuous diagnosis with traits that we all possess to one degree or another. Those who are diagnosed with ADHD have such a high degree of these traits that they have functional impairment in their everyday lives and it results in functional impairment and mental health problems.[1] We also know that underlying ADHD is a multifactorial causality in which genetic and environmental factors interact to create what for every individual is a unique model of vulnerability. At the end of the day, we all carry gene variants associated with ADHD traits and will all – to a greater or lesser extent – be exposed to environmental factors that raise or lower our individual risk. No single gene or environmental factor is necessary or sufficient, and people with ADHD are not qualitatively or distinctly different from people without the diagnosis.[2]

The ADHD diagnosis, just like other psychiatric diagnoses, is essentially only a description of a wide array of symptoms, behaviours, and problems in a person's life. There are no medical tests, blood works, or radiological examinations that unequivocally could prove that you do or don't have the diagnosis. Rather, ADHD is characterized by symptoms within two key domains: *inattentiveness* and *hyperactivity/impulsivity*. For a child to be diagnosed with ADHD, he or she must display at least six of the nine criteria within one or both domains. The mathematically gifted can work out that all possible combinations of these 18 criteria create 116,220 ways in which ADHD can manifest in any one individual. So, if you tell me that you have ADHD, I'll still know very little about you and your life.

My aim in writing this book is to look beyond these diagnostic criteria and describe what it can be like to live with ADHD, as a female and in different stages of life. I'll review what contemporary neuroscience tells us about how the ADHD brain works and give a popular scientific and, I hope, comprehensive presentation of what we currently know about the aetiology and underlying mechanism of ADHD, with a particular focus on how it can manifest in and be experienced by girls and women. It's important, in this context, to point out that what I describe here is based on today's best available scientific knowledge and that I have done my best to simplify quite complex processes and associations. Furthermore, since the first edition of this book was published in Swedish in 2019, there have been some substantial additions to the current scientific literature. Most importantly, Professor Susan Young and colleagues have published a long-awaited, important, and influential expert consensus statement for the identification and treatment of female ADHD across the lifespan.[3] Sometimes, when I read my own text, I get the feeling that we have solved the mystery behind how the ADHD brain works. Nothing could be further from the truth. We are still a long way from understanding exactly how our complex brain works and what happens when something functions differently.

There is a list of references and suggested further reading material at the end of the book for anyone wanting to explore the field in more depth. I specifically recommend the excellent research overview by Professor Young and colleagues from 2020, 'Females with ADHD: An expert consensus statement taking a lifespan approach providing guidance for the identification and treatment of attention-deficit/hyperactivity disorder in girls and women' published in *BMC Psychiatry*.[4] Their selective review of the research literature on ADHD in girls and women provides guidance to improve identification, treatment, and support for girls and women with ADHD across the lifespan.

Notes

1 Larsson *et al.*, 2012
2 Larsson *et al.*, 2013
3 Young *et al.*, 2020
4 Young *et al.*, 2020

Chapter 1

The Background

Social structures

As we become increasingly better at recognizing and describing ADHD, more and more individuals will receive a diagnosis, especially adult women. But why is this? Are we witnessing an ADHD epidemic in older females? Or are we looking at ADHD from a skewed gender perspective? Are there group-level differences in how ADHD is expressed in men and women that have previously been ignored?

Regrettably, we still seem to expect different behaviours from girls and boys, be it at school, at play, or at home. The definition of 'normal' is, in many contexts, quite different for women and men. Perhaps many of us are keener to turn a blind eye to Granddad forgetting his grandchildren's birthdays than Grandma? And perhaps we find it more charming when Dad again packs the wrong gym clothes than when Mum forgets the packed lunch for the school trip? When looking at the diagnostic processes for ADHD, other sex and gender issues emerge. Our diagnostic tools give us little guidance on how gender and culture differences affect how symptoms are expressed and interpreted.

Could this be because a majority of the children on whom the diagnostic criteria are based were European and American boys? Or could it be due to a gloomier message: that adults simply take a more disparaging view of girls who don't fit the norm?

'Flickprojektet' (The Girl Project), initiated by a leading group of researchers including Svenny Kopp and Professor Christopher Gillberg in Gothenburg back in 1999, spent several years monitoring girls between three and 18 years of age with various neurodevelopmental disorders, including ADHD. Their report showed that even if parents are quick to notice their daughter's problems, most of the girls with ADHD will be overlooked in school. In addition, it's not until years after the first appeal for help that daughters obtain the correct diagnosis and explanatory model for their problems.

They also found that girls with ADHD, even if they may be invisible to others, by no means suffer less or have fewer problems. On the contrary, they have, besides ADHD, many other psychiatric diagnoses and, in many cases, severe functional impairments.[1]

The bitter truth is, when compared to boys, girls with ADHD receive less attention in school, are less popular among teachers, and have fewer friends. Because of that, girls with ADHD – who can have serious learning difficulties, psychosocial challenges, and psychiatric comorbidities as well – receive less support than boys with the same diagnosis.

Girls and women with ADHD are overlooked because they do not fit into the classic ADHD stereotype of the hyperactive boy. Unlike 'disruptive' boys, girls with ADHD are more often regarded as shy, reserved, and compliant. Their constant struggle to hide their difficulties can, paradoxically, hinder them from receiving correct diagnoses and accommodations.

After all, a 'well-adjusted' girl usually displays nothing of the disruptiveness and impulsivity that we expect of someone with ADHD.

However, many girls and women realize early on in life that something is different about them. Sometimes they seek help, but more often they decide to attempt to conform to society's expectations and appear normal. Turning feelings of inadequacy inwards, they're often burdened with shame and guilt. And as long as they finish school without causing trouble, they likely do not receive a referral for assessment and treatment. But just like for the boys, each month and year that passes without a diagnosis and a correct explanatory model increases the risk of underperforming or even failing in school, of emotional and relationship problems, and of feelings of inadequacy and alienation. Also worth noting is that intellectually gifted girls with ADHD seem to be even less likely to be recognized, and the delay until diagnosis increases along with the level of their intellectual capacity.[2]

In an ADHD assessment, teams often try to determine whether someone exhibits a pattern of academic failure, externalizing, or impulsive behaviour. However, since these common displays of ADHD are less typical in girls, they tend to function longer until the external demands on self-efficacy and independency escalate. More typically, girls seek help for internalizing problems such as anxiety, depression, eating disorders, and self-harm, as their former coping strategies no longer suffice, threatening to unmask their difficulties. Girls, as a group, also mature psychosocially earlier than boys, knowing at an earlier age what is expected from them and how to behave in different contexts. This makes it even more important that we compare them with their female peers rather than with same-aged boys.

We know now that ADHD is a diagnosis that most individuals won't grow out of: research indicates that between 50 to 75 per cent of children with ADHD will experience impairing symptoms into adulthood and across their entire lifespan.[3] Even though it's still much more common for boys to be diagnosed with ADHD, by the time we start looking at the number of adult men and women with a diagnosis, the gender difference in incidence begins to even out.

Biology

Keeping in mind that all individuals are equal and should be treated as equals, there are nonetheless important differences between males and females. From a biological perspective, the two sexes differ in terms of our bodies and the physiology of their organs. The brain is no exception. To fully embrace the notion that women are more than just slightly smaller men, we need to understand how these sex differences arise and how they impact what we do, think, and need.

At the moment of fertilization, our biological sex is determined by the lucky X or Y chromosome bearing sperm that first manages to penetrate the egg membrane. Fairly soon after fertilization, the growing girl or boy embryo will start organizing its cells into clusters forming the body's various organs. At this stage, among much else, the female and male gonad buds appear. The male Y chromosome produces a protein that induces the sex cells of the male embryo to produce testosterone. In the absence of a Y chromosome, as in the case of female embryos carrying two X chromosomes, these cells will develop into oestrogen-producing follicle cells that steer the formation of ovaries, uterus, and the other female sex organs.

The two different sex hormones, testosterone and oestrogen, will have a profound influence on the structure and function of the foetal, child, and adult bodily organs. In the presence of testosterone, a boy develops; in the absence of this hormone, a girl develops.

The rudimentary structure of what will become our nervous system is, in effect, laid down in tandem with the establishment of our sex. The developing nervous system is affected differently by the overarching hormonal system that has been activated – or not, in the case of the female embryo. No hormonal signals are needed for girls to continue developing along the basic blueprint, and the ovaries remain dormant until they receive signals from the pituitary gland to start producing hormones during puberty. In other words, male and female brains are organized differently. At group level, men's brains are about 10 per cent larger than women's. However, the saying 'size doesn't matter' is particularly true when it comes to the brain. We no longer believe that brain volume is the main cause of the group-level differences in behaviour, muscle strength, and susceptibility for certain brain disorders. We do know, however, that there are other salient differences, again at group level, between how the connections within and between different brain regions are organized in men and women.[4]

Some of these structural differences are thought to be related to corresponding differences in their function. Men, for example, have more developed connections *within* each brain hemisphere (between the posterior and anterior parts), while women have stronger connections between the left and right parts of the brain. Generally speaking, the male brain will have an advantage when processing spatial information and boys will, on a group level, find it easier than their female coevals to coordinate their movements in response to different sensory impressions. Abundant connections *between* the cerebral hemispheres, however, make it easier for girls, again on a group level, to understand and process complex situations, enabling them to adapt their behaviour to different social contexts.[5] On average, girls and women will perform better at tasks that demand linguistic and social faculties.[6] These earlier and more advanced social functions may, paradoxically, be one reason why we overlook girls with ADHD. They simply find it easier to understand and adapt to what is expected of them socially at a younger age.

All in all, there are decisive differences between how male and female brains are constructed and how they operate. Of course, it's a simplification to say that a certain brain will behave in a certain way. It is important to bear in mind that there will always be far greater differences between two single individuals than what we can find between two groups. Therefore, there are lots of girls who are super-talented at football, parkour, and maths, as there are, of course, many boys who are extremely socially developed early in life and find almost nothing in common with the stereotypical ADHD boy. All the complicated psychological functions that constitute a person's behaviour in a given situation are, at the end of the day, different combinations of individual biosocial prerequisites, previous life experiences, cultural influences, societal expectations, and unknown variables impossible to quantify and comprehend.

The history of ADHD

When reading or hearing about ADHD in the media, it's easy to get the impression that this diagnosis is a modern-age phenomenon that everyone experiences a bit of once in a while. The first key message of this book is that few things could be further from the truth. ADHD is a valid and reliable medical disorder and, if made after a careful and thorough assessment, an accurate psychiatric diagnosis. More importantly, for most people with ADHD, the diagnosis entails a lifelong disability. I would also like to claim that the diagnosis is by no means a modern figment:

> Every humming fly, every shadow, every sound, the memory of old stories will draw him off his task to other imaginations. Even his own imagination entertains him with a thousand minor subjects. (Melchior Adam Weikard, 1775)

This passage, found in a German medical textbook from 1775, describes the psychiatric disorder that back then was called *Attentio Volubilis*. As far as I'm aware, it's the earliest reference in medical literature to what we today know of as ADHD. According to the German physician and philosopher Weikard, 'an inauspicious childhood environment could render nerve fibres soft and delicate, impairing the ability to maintain constant attention'.[8]

Besides suggestions for therapeutic strategies – which on the current knowledge seem as unethical as they are absurd – such as keeping an affected child in dark isolation, forcing them to take cold baths, or medicating with milk, acids, and spices, Weikard also proposed many things that concur with modern evidence-based methods. For instance, he recommended exercise such as gymnastics and horseback riding, arguing that physical activities often made these children more settled and better able to concentrate.[9] Not long afterwards, in 1798, the Scottish-born physician Alexander Crichton noted that attention deficits in children and teenagers were often congenital and associated with other mental and physical problems. This, too, is in line with our current view of neurodevelopmental disorders and common comorbidities associated with ADHD. Crichton, as Weikard had before him, described the core symptoms of ADHD in a way that almost fully corresponds to the diagnostic criteria used in the current diagnostic manual, DSM-5 (see p.26).[10]

Perhaps the best known and most quoted historical description of ADHD was published in the *Goulstonian Lectures* 1902 by Sir George Frederic Still, England's first professor of paediatric medicine. The lectures consisted of accounts of 43 children struggling with serious problems of inattention and self-control. Still described these children as 'hyperactive, aggressive, defiant, resistant to discipline, as well as excessively emotional or passionate'. The children, he said, had a 'defect in inhibitory volition', which he assumed had a biological aetiology. A need for immediate gratification was consistent in these children, who, according to Still, 'could not seem to learn from the consequences of their actions although their intellect was normal'.[11]

ADHD or ADD? The different diagnostic manuals

Over the years, the description of ADHD and ADD (attention deficit disorder) has changed and developed along with increased clinical experiences and advances in research. New knowledge and understanding have been gradually accumulated and organized into manuals to help physicians systematize disorders and diagnoses. Systemization is important since it enables physicians and healthcare professionals to deliver treatments corresponding to specific conditions. Moreover, a systematic organization of different symptoms and syndromes provides a common language for healthcare workers when discussing their patients' various difficulties.

Two different diagnostic systems have been in use since the 1950s: the *International Statistical Classification of Diseases and Related Health Problems* (ICD) and the *Diagnostic and Statistical Manual of Mental Disorders* (DSM). The ICD and DSM are used in parallel and have, in the past, been mutually consistent. But the latest version of DSM (DSM-5), published in 2013, contains some important additions and alterations as compared to the currently used ICD version, the ICD-10. These differences have practical consequences for neurodevelopmental disorders, including ADHD, that we will be returning to later in the book.

Consequently, the ADHD diagnosis has changed across the different revised versions of the two diagnostic manuals. In the first edition to include neurodevelopmental conditions, the DSM-III from 1980, all forms of ADHD were referred to as 'attention deficit disorder' (ADD), to which a qualification could be added if someone had ADD 'with hyperactivity'. In the fourth edition, DSM-IV, published in 1994, three different subtypes of ADHD appeared for the first time: inattentive, hyperactive, and combined form.

The distinction between ADHD and ADD has been fluid over the years. For example, impulsivity was regarded as part of inattentiveness in DSM-III, while the next edition had it as belonging to the group of hyperactive symptoms. Consequently, many researchers and experienced clinicians argue that the distinction between ADHD and ADD may be problematic and shouldn't be given too much weight.

ADHD symptoms can vary widely throughout a lifetime, and hyperactivity and impulsivity often become less salient during adulthood. Thus, we rarely see a grown woman climbing over furniture in a meeting room or physically launching herself at an opponent during a heated argument. This doesn't necessarily mean that she has grown out of her ADHD or that she's gone from ADHD to ADD. The hyperactivity can instead have 'colonized' the body as a constant state of inner restlessness and anxiety, not obvious to others around her.

To some extent, the difference in prevalence of ADHD in girls versus boys can be explained by the types of studies we have in front of us. For instance, studies observe greater differences between girls' and boys' ADHD symptoms when examining a selection of patients at a psychiatric clinic rather than samples from the general population. This may partly be explained by girls needing to exhibit more pronounced problems than boys for a referral to a clinic for ADHD. This in turn may lead to boys assessed for ADHD being 'normal boys with ADHD', while girls assessed for the same diagnosis not being 'normal girls with ADHD', but rather girls with more serious problems – that is, 'abnormal girls with ADHD'.

A large meta-analysis, combining information from several smaller studies, suggests that girls with ADHD exhibit less hyperactive behaviour than boys.[12] However, the fact that girls and women as a group display fewer motor-hyperactive symptoms doesn't necessarily mean that all girls have ADD and all boys have ADHD. And, most importantly, there is no decisive difference in the suffering and disability that ADHD entails for girls and boys, regardless of study design.

In the 2013 edition of the diagnostic manual, DSM-5, the diagnostic criteria for ADHD have been adapted to better describe typical symptoms at different stages of life. Adolescents and adults over the age of 17 need to fulfil five criteria rather than six from either domain. Additionally, the symptoms should be presented before the age of 12, instead of seven. Whereas previously, someone could only be diagnosed with either ADHD or autism, it's now recognized that both conditions can be present in the same person and this is fairly common. Furthermore, the recent edition of DSM focuses less on the different subtypes and more on the underlying presentation of ADHD – that is, different proxies for the difficulties that many with ADHD describe in their everyday lives. We will get back to these different neurocognitive displays in several parts of this book.

How common is ADHD?

Looking at the quantitative rather than qualitative view of the ADHD diagnosis, as well as understanding the normal distribution of common traits and characteristics associated with ADHD, it becomes relatively easy to assess approximately how many individuals there are who statistically 'should' fill the diagnosis in a given population. Indeed, international research shows that 5 to 9 per cent of all children worldwide display impairments with concentration, hyperactivity, and impulsivity required to meet the criteria for an ADHD diagnosis. In adults, the corresponding number is about 2 per cent.[13] However, although we are fairly certain of the 'true prevalence' of ADHD, the diagnosis is more widespread in certain countries and regions. There may be many possible explanations for this.

Some prevalence measures will derive from studies among children and adults in a clinical setting. A larger proportion of individuals who are referred for or themselves seek help for psychiatric symptoms will meet the criteria of an ADHD diagnosis than those measured in the general population. People who have not yet been diagnosed with ADHD may also seek help for other problems, since comorbidity is a common feature of the condition. Thus, one must take into account what kind of setting prevalence estimates are drawn from.

The fact that ADHD is more prevalent in certain countries can also be attributable to the diagnostic manual used. For example, the ICD diagnostic system, common in Europe, gives rise to fewer diagnosed individuals than DSM, the system more common in the USA. This is because the DSM system is devised in such a way that makes the diagnostic criteria easier to fulfil.

Another important factor for local differences in ADHD prevalence is the fact that neurodevelopmental disorders never exist in a vacuum. Someone's ADHD symptoms may cause varying degrees of impairments depending on other individual characteristics, the external environment, cultural expectations, and the level of accommodations made by others. The diagnostic process per se may also influence how many ADHD diagnoses are rendered. Relying solely on screening forms and self-ratings will give rise to a large number of 'false positives' since these instruments are designed to gather all individuals displaying problems in a certain area. Some screen positives will have ADHD, but many of them will have other reasons for their symptoms. We all know that hyperactivity, impulsivity, and inattention can be caused by many different factors and situations. Furthermore, we all have some degree of impulsivity and different ability to concentrate in different contexts. It's only when the problems become serious and disabling over time and in multiple settings that we consider an ADHD diagnosis.

Widespread fear that ADHD diagnoses are too common finds little support in the scientific literature.[14] If anything, most studies suggest that the increase in ADHD diagnoses is mainly due to better recognition of the difficulties with which people with ADHD struggle. Particularly in girls and women there have been, and still are, many undetected cases. Yet unpublished data from my research group shows that, on average, it takes five years longer for a girl with ADHD to be diagnosed correctly compared to a same-aged boy – years that are dogged by endless suffering, both for her and her loved ones.

What is ADHD?

ADHD belongs to a category of psychiatric diagnosis labelled neurodevelopmental disorders. The 'neuro' part derives from the fact that these conditions were first described and treated by neurologists – physicians who specialize in disorders of the nervous system – who first observed that children with different kinds of neurological disorders, such as epilepsy, congenital malformations, cerebral palsy, or different genetic syndromes, often also had behavioural impairments. For many years, ADHD was believed to only manifest in children. Adult psychiatrists were not trained to detect and follow these problems once the children had grown up.

In this book, we will look beyond the diagnostic criteria of ADHD in girls and women; nevertheless, I would still like to briefly summarize the approach towards diagnosing ADHD – or not diagnosing it.

To fulfil the criteria for an ADHD diagnosis, a child or adult needs to experience and exhibit 'persistent problems of sustained attention and/or impulsiveness and hyperactivity'. These (ADHD) symptoms must have caused lifelong impairments and suffering within multiple domains[15] and need to be described before the age of 12. Therefore, it's not particularly easy, as some people claim, to receive an ADHD diagnosis.

The assessment team, consisting of a specialized psychiatrist and psychologist, conducts a detailed investigation for evidence, experiences, behaviours, situations, and impairments attributable to underlying difficulties to sustain attention and control activity levels and impulses. Since everyone will find it difficult to concentrate, think ahead, plan, and organize in times of crisis, anxiety, fever, starvation, or following excessive substance use, it becomes important to rule out the possibility that the problems could be better explained by a temporary condition or a separate physiological or psychiatric disorder.

As of today, more and more girls and women are being diagnosed with ADHD. For many of them, it will be the first time that they are given a clear explanation for their lifelong experiences of abnormality, alienation, low self-esteem, social failure, or psychiatric comorbidity. Undiagnosed and untreated ADHD will cause personal suffering and private impairments, in school or at work, at a high economic cost for the individual themselves, their families, and society in general.[16] ADHD is also associated with an increased risk of both physical and psychiatric comorbidities. It leaves people prone to accidents and destructive alcohol and drug use, and in some more severe cases, can lead to criminality, suicidality, and substance use disorders.

To be specific, our current understanding of ADHD tells us that people who meet the criteria for this controversial diagnosis have a life expectancy about ten years shorter than those who have no diagnosis.[17] So talking about ADHD as something you can 'have a bout of' or as a 'superpower' isn't just demeaning and offensive, it's also very far from the truth. ADHD is not a condition that we could or should sweep under the rug.

If we agree that ADHD is a serious condition that, once identified and treated, has a good prognosis, then we should also consider how knowledge, early detection, proper accommodations, and evidence-based treatment can prevent much of what could risk affecting or even disabling children and adults with ADHD. There is a strong international consensus that ADHD must be assessed, diagnosed, and treated if adverse consequences and personal suffering are to be avoided.[18]

Perhaps the term ADHD per se is part of the problem of why we seem to find it so difficult to take this lifelong and sometimes life-threatening disability seriously. The name *attention deficit and hyperactivity disorder* is itself actually quite misleading. You may get the impression that it's just a case of pulling yourself together and getting a grip of your life. However, when someone with ADHD describes their daily existence, another truth emerges. Additionally, physicians who regularly meet with children and adults with ADHD tend to take this diagnosis quite seriously indeed. It's not just a problem that we lose children in accidents, teenagers to suicide, and young adults in road accidents; ADHD takes years out of the lives of those affected across the entire lifespan.

Still, not too long ago, it was thought that someone with ADHD was out of the danger zone once they had made it through their tempestuous teens. Unfortunately, that isn't the case. Growing out of adolescence, many adults with ADHD keep living as if there is no tomorrow, and this will have dire consequences. In the next chapter, we'll be looking more closely at why people with ADHD so easily fall into this tendency and why research shows that living without the proper ADHD diagnosis and treatment is living a life at risk of accidents and trauma, failure in school, alcohol and drug addiction, self-harm, traffic accidents, employment issues, obesity, chronic physical conditions, and loneliness. Those with the highest risk of developing lifestyle problems are also the ones who find it the hardest to assimilate the support and therapy that society devises to mitigate their health problems.

So, what is ADHD – really?

I hope that it is already clear that ADHD is more than just problematic inattentiveness and hyperactivity. Sadly, our instruments for detecting these difficulties are quite poor, especially for adults and, above all, for women. This can partly be attributed to the fact that our diagnostic systems are restricted to measuring the behavioural output of the diagnostic criteria. What many people living with ADHD are aware of, and what researchers and clinicians have long known, is that ADHD is much more than its 18 diagnostic criteria. To better understand what ADHD is really all about, you may want to take a closer look at some underlying neuropsychological mechanisms of the diagnosis.

1. Difficulties with executive attention

The letter A in ADHD stands for Attention. Perhaps one reason why we don't understand the serious nature of ADHD is that we don't fully grasp the importance of attention. As humans, we have a unique ability to calculate the future in relation to the past and present and adjust our behaviour to later, hypothetical events. The ability to remember what we're doing, to keep future goals in mind, and recognize the steps to achieve them is a vital part of our attention. This is often referred to as the working memory. Our executive functions make it possible for us to plan, organize, and synchronize all the different bits and pieces that need to be set in motion, at the right time and in the right place, for us to achieve our future goals.

When we work towards the future, much of what happens around us in the meantime can distract or divert our attention from what we're aiming to achieve. If you have ADHD, however, your attention may be so fragile that you lose sight of your long-term goal. Instead of finding your way back to the path to your goal, you're distracted. Executive attention enables us, in competition with millions of distractions, to perform everything from the simplest everyday chore to more advanced mental calculations – to understand what we're reading, follow a conversation or a film, receive instructions or to give them to our child. When ADHD is defined as impaired executive attention causing difficulties preparing for the future, it becomes easier to grasp the scale of the condition and what it entails for those living with it. Due to impaired executive attention, ADHD becomes something that impinges on everything required for a healthy and prosperous life.

2. Difficulties controlling and regulating cognitive and motivational processes

The diagnostic manual contains many descriptions of hyperactive and impulsive behaviour. The problem is that overt hyperactivity is less common in females as a group. Moreover, it wanes with age and so is rarer in adults. The diagnostic instruments at large fail to capture many of the consequences of cognitive and emotional impulsivity and motivation deficits – functions that help us pause and think before we do or say something. People struggling in this regard often end up in a pattern of disjointed and disorganized activities that may lead to feelings of chaos and many uncompleted projects.

Many with ADHD do not describe motor hyperactivity as their greatest problem; more often the difficulty controlling thoughts and ideas is perceived as more impairing for adults. Diagnostic manuals, however, lack appropriate measures for this 'cognitive and motivational impulsivity'. Still, these poorly described deficiencies can have serious consequences. We can take social relationships as an example. Social interaction is often about being able to control and adapt our behaviour and curb our desire for immediate gratification. If we cannot hold back on our immediate impulse to say or do things in a social setting, this will likely have consequences. Thus, many of the core difficulties described by people with ADHD, such as making and keeping friendships, engaging in risk-taking behaviours, and having work-life failures can be understood in terms of motivational deficits and cognitive hyperactivity or impulsivity.

Moreover, living with ADHD often makes it harder to sustain motivation long enough to endure temporary adversity or discomfort. This makes it difficult to achieve more long-term goals even if you have the sufficient executive functions to plan and organize them. Conversely, it is also quite common that certain tasks will feel so super-motivating that it is close to impossible to stop doing them. With ADHD, you may be able to stay perfectly focused for extremely long periods. Unfortunately, the focus is often not always on what is necessary to be done, giving outsiders the impression that focus is a self-serving decision. Comments such as 'I've seen how long you can concentrate on your painting, weeding, or playing accordion' or, 'You're lazy and just doing what you want to do, not what you have to,' are no doubt common in families of people with ADHD. As renowned sage and world famous ADHD researcher Professor Russell Barkley elegantly puts it: ADHD is not about knowing what you should do, but rather doing what you should do.

The ADHD assessment

The purpose of a neuropsychological assessment is to find the best explanatory model for recurrent everyday difficulties and impairments. Besides certain important neuropsychological tests, the investigation is based on information collected by skilled and experienced clinicians the individual knows and trusts – a team of psychiatrists, psychologists, special needs teachers, physiotherapists, and sometimes occupational therapists.

A proper assessment can only be done if the family, child, or adult is willing to offer the information necessary for the right conclusions to be drawn. It's a collaboration between the patient, significant others, and the investigative team. The most important parts of the puzzle are held by the patient and their family, with the team itself working to fit the pieces together to create a full picture. The final product is an individual functional map to which the patient and their family can relate and start navigating towards.

As described earlier, psychiatric diagnoses are really just names given to groups of symptoms, behaviours, and problems experienced by an individual. Because diagnostic labels have and will continue to change over the years as our understanding of the underlying mechanisms does, it's important to gain a thorough description of the problems experienced and the everyday difficulties they cause.

If you tell me that you have ADHD, I still know almost nothing about you. It takes a unique map of your strengths and vulnerabilities for a diagnosis to be useful. In other words, an assessment is all but worthless if its aim is to just state whether someone has or does not have ADHD.

A well-conducted ADHD assessment should contain as many data points as possible. In the case of a child, the assessment team talks to parents, grandparents, teachers, and other adults who know the child and their family. Both children and adults can find it difficult to articulate things they don't normally talk about, which makes school visits and observations of potential problems and difficulties in the child's natural environment key.

In the case of an adult, the assessment team always collects collateral information from both past and present acquaintances and friends, including those from childhood. The experienced difficulties must have been present throughout the person's life, with an onset before the age of 12, to be consistent with ADHD. Sometimes this can't be ascertained if family or friends from childhood aren't available or allowed to be involved. In such cases, the investigative team must be creative and find other sources of information.

For many people, a sound, well-conducted neuropsychological assessment is a therapeutic, healing experience in itself. At best, you gain insight into and understanding of why different aspects of your life have been so hard, and why you might have struggled more than your peers. For many, the assessment and following diagnosis marks the beginning of a new journey towards greater self-esteem and a more balanced life.

Screening and self-reports

The self-rating scales and questionnaires found online or those used by healthcare services are designed to identify a shared set of symptoms that characterize the diagnosis or signs of the disorder. The screening forms used by healthcare professionals and in research are often carefully checked and tested to reliably and effectively capture everyone at risk for a certain diagnosis. However, it's important to remember that many of those identified through screening will not meet the criteria for the specific disorder at all. They may just have more of the symptoms in question than others, or they may have symptoms better explained by a different condition.

The next step in a proper assessment is to find those who genuinely meet the criteria for the diagnosis. There are different methods of doing this; however, when it comes to psychiatric diagnoses, we can't rely on invasive or purely objective tests like blood work or radiology. Instead, we use diagnostic interviews, personal accounts, and collateral information from significant others. We can increase the accuracy of our assessment by using different psychological test and data collection methods.

As discussed earlier, the ADHD diagnosis is based on 18 different criteria divided into two domains (inattention and hyperactivity/impulsivity). When a child meets six or more criteria from either or both domains and has debilitating problems with several aspects of life caused by these symptoms, we can consider whether the problems are best described within the context of an ADHD diagnosis. Young people over the age of 17 and adults need to meet at least five of the criteria in one or both symptom groups.

The ADHD language – a phrase dictionary

Thankfully, through diagnostic criteria we have effectively operationalized symptoms and descriptions that otherwise may seem vague or hard to pin down. But this systematic approach is not altogether without issues. More specifically, the existing screening and diagnostic tools may be particularly problematic for girls and women. This is because most assessment has been based on how ADHD manifests in boys and men. Many men and women also often find the diagnostic criteria too one-dimensional and simplistic to do justice to the nuances of what they struggle with in their everyday life.

After encountering many individuals with the same diagnosis, certain patterns will inevitably emerge. These are patterns that, despite myriad interpersonal differences, constantly recur in the stories and testimonies shared. The ADHD language, developed by UK psychologists Kobus van Rensburg and Mohammad Arif, is woven by thin, recurring threads from the stories of adults with ADHD they have met over the years.[19] The process of assessment and treatment of ADHD can be highly enriched by asking directly about symptoms of ADHD, and listening attentively for indirect cues.

So, what are girls and women really saying when they try to explain their problems originating from the two core domains of ADHD: inattention and hyperactivity/impulsivity?

In the ADHD language, what the psychiatrist refers to as symptoms of inattentiveness may sound like this:

- 'When I read stuff, I always jump around in the text, and I lose myself and miss important details. I often have to read it all over again, so even though I try to hurry, it still takes me longer.'
- 'I write long lists to help me remember what I must do. It calms me down in some strange way. But then I never follow them and end up writing new ones.'
- 'I hate deadlines; they stress me out completely. But I need them because I have to put some serious pressure on myself or nothing happens.'

- 'I often leave the planning and organizing to my husband. It's so hard to know in what order to do stuff in anyway. It's nice when he just tells me what I need to do.'
- 'I've given up trying to understand anything at the first attempt. I always have to ask again anyway.'
- 'I really do try to keep up, but I'm constantly distracted by my own thoughts and all the fun things that pop up in my head. It's like my mind never shuts up.'
- 'My children tease me because I always ask them if they have seen my phone, glasses, or laptop.'
- 'I'm really exhausted just by trying to keep the basic things in my head, to try to get some order in all the chaos in the outside world.'

If the psychiatrist says that someone shows symptoms of hyperactivity and impulsivity, framing those experiences in the ADHD language can sound like this:

- 'Even when I want to be careful, I rush to get things done. I may miss a few details, but I'm almost always the one who finishes first.'
- 'I always want to be on the move. The worst thing for me is when nothing happens. I'm sooooooo easily bored and sometimes I pick a fight just to cure the boredom of things.'
- 'People get stressed out and nervous around me; they say I'm always fiddling with my hands, chewing my hair, or bouncing my legs.'
- 'Other people say I go at "top speed" all the time, but I usually just feel completely exhausted.'
- 'I get that it's hard to watch movies with me, as I keep leaving my seat to get stuff, check my mobile, go to the toilet. I need to do something else to be able to concentrate on the film.'

- 'I'm allergic to slow pace; I get bored so easily. I'd do almost anything to avoid being bored.'
- 'Other people say I'm disruptive and always have to get involved, but I hate it when things are all quiet. That makes me zone out and almost fall asleep.'
- 'I never feel calm and peaceful inside. It's much better when there's a lot going on, so that the outside matches what's going on inside.'
- 'It's so unfair; I really need to rest and relax but can never find the inner peace to do it, even if I have the opportunity.'
- 'Other people are so slow; they drag everything out to absurdity. I mean, can't we just get started?'
- 'I notice that other people get annoyed when I finish their sentences, but I already know what they're going to say, and they never get to the point.'
- 'If I don't say what I think straight away, it's gone. And I'm left with a horrible feeling that I've forgotten something.'
- 'I just can't stop myself; when I think about all the risks I have taken, a chill runs down my spine.'

Another way to identify typical characteristics of ADHD is to read between the lines of what women with ADHD say about themselves:

- 'I've always known that I'm different. I get so upset when people don't understand that and try to explain to me that "everyone feels like that".'
- 'I often forget to eat. But once I start, I can't stop. It's shameful to be an adult still struggling with binge eating.'
- 'It wasn't that I didn't understand things at school. It's just it was never clear how it all fits together.'

- 'I behave like a teenager when it comes to feelings and emotions.'
- 'My soul and body are worn out; I just want someone to sedate me.'
- 'I've had loads of different jobs but always get fed up when others try to tell me what to do.'
- 'I've probably hurt a lot of people over the years. I feel ashamed of so much I've said and done.'
- 'I need to take something to feel normal...'
- 'I was called the night-owl as a baby. My thoughts still keep me awake at night and then I can never get up in the morning.'
- 'Sometimes I hesitate to start even fun things because I know I'll get manic and overdo it.'
- 'I've had so many diagnoses through life, but none really fitted.'
- 'The treatment helped in some ways, but to be honest I just replaced one problematic behaviour with another.'
- 'I realize people don't trust me. I don't trust myself either.'

In my role as a psychiatrist, I'm also in a position to ask what sort of thing women with ADHD hear from other people. They often tell me that others often tell them things like:

- 'Come on, everyone thinks cleaning and paying bills is boring.'
- 'Why is there always so much drama in your life?'
- 'But I've already explained this to you several times.'
- 'Hello, earth calling! Can you please listen to me when I'm talking to you?'
- 'You're hopeless; you asked me where your phone was two minutes ago.'
- 'Please, let me finish what I was trying to say.'
- 'I know you can do it if you just try a little harder.'

- 'What on earth were you thinking? We've talked about this...'
- 'I can't deal with your excuses any more. You're just not willing to change, or you wouldn't still be doing this.'

Notes

1   Kopp & Gillberg, 2003; Kopp *et al.*, 2010
2   Milioni *et al.*, 2017
3   Franke *et al.*, 2018
4   Bale & Epperson, 2017
5   Ingalhalikar *et al.*, 2014
6   Gur *et al.*, 2012
7   Barkley & Peters, 2012
8   Barkley & Peters, 2012
9   Doyle, 2004
10 Barkley, 2006
11 Hasson & Fine, 2012; Gershon, 2002
12 Kessler *et al.*, 2006
13 Polanczyk *et al.*, 2014
14 Faraone *et al.*, 2015
15 Nilsson & Nilsson-Lundmark, 2013
16 Barkley & Fischer, 2019
17 Coghill *et al.*, 2017; Thapar & Cooper, 2016
18 van Rensburg & Arif, 2019

Chapter 2

ADHD and the Brain

About the brain

It could hardly have escaped anyone that the brain is a fiercely complex organ. The human brain is comprised of roughly one hundred billion nerve cells (neurons), each of which has a couple of thousand connections to neighbouring neurons. These connections, or synapses, convey information from one neuron to another via electrical and chemical signals.

Thanks to brain-imaging techniques, we are learning more about how our thoughts, emotions and behaviours are linked to processes in different parts of the brain. Each individual brain is wired through unique circuits and in a constant state of flux as it responds to how life experiences shape our behaviours and personality traits.

Even though more advanced neuroscience lies beyond the scope of this book, it's this very science that has helped us understand what happens when something in these circuits fail, or when the synapses don't work as they should. Neuroscience gives us more insight into human behaviour and differences, both at group and individual level.

The chemical substances neurons use for communication

are called neurotransmitters. When an electrical signal from one cell reaches another, the neuron releases these substances that in turn affect how the cell behaves. When these signals are repeated, the connections between the cells are reinforced and the neurons change shape, creating new synapses and routes of communication. This process is, put very simply, the basis of how we learn from experience, form memories, and shape routines.

The frontal lobes – there is a tomorrow

Many with ADHD will tell us that many of their problems are caused by decisions made from inadequate information or by saying thoughtless things in the heat of the moment. Impulsivity can be the root of many serious problems in ADHD. Today, we understand impulsivity as a deficit in the higher functions of the brain, more specifically in the frontal lobes, which have poor control over evolutionary older parts of the nervous system like the reward systems.

Our brain, like all other parts of the body, has developed greatly throughout evolution. While we share many of the older parts of our brain with other 'lower' lifeforms, hundreds of millions of years ago, as vertebrates we began to evolve the precursors of more advanced brain structures.[1]

The brain's frontal lobes control and bring order to the multitude of competing external signals from the world around us. Fully developed and functional frontal lobes enable us to adjust and, in many cases, inhibit impulses, allowing our actions to become purposeful and appropriate. Humans, unlike other animals, can think and plan for the future. Humans can, for example, imagine the outcome to different sequences of events depending on alternative actions. Put simply, the frontal lobes control our executive attention and regulate our responses to various emotions and impressions.

Every day, we face challenges and problems that have no preconceived or clear solution. In these situations, the frontal lobes cooperate with other brain areas to identify and devise innovative solutions. The frontal lobes also factor in new information that may clash with previous experiences. Based on this complex information, the frontal lobes choose the most appropriate path to achieve our desires and goals.

As we age from infancy into young adulthood, the different areas of our brains develop, roughly speaking, from the neck to the forehead. Consequently, the frontal lobes will be the last brain structure to fully mature. In fact, the frontal lobes reach full functionality in most around the age of 20 or 25 (this is reached earlier in girls/women than in boys/men).[2]

In other words, once fully mature, the frontal lobes will act as the symphony conductor, making sure that the entire cerebral orchestra plays in synchrony. Your frontal lobes account for the adult, wise, reflective part of you, telling you to think again before unleashing more primitive impulses.

The reward systems – pleasure at any cost

It's common for people with ADHD to say that they find it hard to resist immediate temptations, or that they fall for transitory, short-lived pleasures at the cost of their long-term goals and desires.

Long before the advent of homo sapiens and the frontal

lobes, there were what the popular science often refers to as more primitive reward systems. These subcortical brain areas have been left relatively intact through evolution, even while the rest of the brain has evolved and changed dramatically. Though it might be surprising, there's very little difference between the reward systems of humans and those of cats or mice. Yet the fact that these systems have persevered throughout evolution gives us a clue as to how crucial they are to our survival.

Our motivation and reward systems help us control our behaviour and steer us towards what is advantageous for us at any particular moment. In fact, the activity in these brain areas gives us the means to take instant decisions, here and now, increasing the chances of our own – and our species' – survival.

But the reward systems are not particularly reliable and useful for navigating towards more long-term goals. For this, we need the more analytical cognition – the planning capacity and consequence awareness of our frontal lobes. We know that people with ADHD react more intensely when their reward system is activated. Therefore, they may struggle to put off instant gratification in the interest of greater gains later, even though they know intellectually that they ought to act more circumspectly.

Dopamine, a neurotransmitter described below, is a key player in the reward system as well as in the frontal lobes and has an important role in ADHD. Today, most neuroscientists agree that dysregulated dopamine levels are one of the underpinning mechanisms explaining why individuals with ADHD have less control over their reward system. It's not as simple as too much or too little dopamine. Instead, most current hypotheses suggest that the ADHD brain has a different way of utilizing and reacting to dopamine release.

The basal ganglia – the brain's autopilot

Most people think of Parkinson's disease when they hear about the basal ganglia and dopamine. There's good reason to, as both dopamine and these structures are also involved in motion and movements. In the case of ADHD, however, it's also the interaction between the basal ganglia and other brain areas – including the frontal lobes – that functions differently.

Our everyday life consists of a myriad of seemingly simple, repetitive tasks. However, viewed from the brain's perspective, all these tasks involve an unimaginable amount of complicated and abstract steps that need to be carried out in a certain order to result in a preferred action. The number of ways we can choose to attain the same goals is mindboggling, and the basal ganglia gather information, filter through, and automate (commit to memory) the behaviours that are most effective.

The brain demands a high amount of energy to complete tasks – consuming some 20 per cent of your everyday energy intake – so it's no mystery that our body wants us to conserve energy. One way for the brain to operate more efficiently is to create rules and routines for things that we do often, so that we can devote our energy to things that are new, unknown, and possibly dangerous.

We can barely conceive of the sheer number of repetitive tasks we accomplish every day. We operate on autopilot and, for this to work, the frontal lobes and the basal ganglia need to agree on the essential information to attain our long-term goals. Thus, the basal ganglia allow us to 'automate' our everyday tasks, instead of constantly reinventing the wheel.

The automation of everyday activities seems to be more difficult with ADHD. A suboptimal communication between the frontal lobes and the basal ganglia may be one reason why so many with ADHD find it completely exhausting to perform even the most routine tasks to any degree of satisfaction.

The cerebellum – small but no less important

Many children and adults with ADHD report difficulties with coordination and motor activity, leaving them feeling clumsy and awkward, inept at learning certain movements, or constantly bumping into or dropping things.

The cerebellum (Latin for 'small brain') coordinates movement and balance based on our surroundings, making sure that signals from the brain reach the correct organ or muscle. It also connects to the frontal lobes, the reward systems, and the basal ganglia, playing an important role in emotional control, the imprinting of memories, and the cognitive faculties involved in learning. Recent research also suggests that the cerebellum may be involved in symptoms manifesting as impulsivity and obsessiveness in obsessive and compulsive disorder (OCD) as well as habit formation and executive functions, commonly seen in people with ADHD.[3]

Even though there is as yet limited research on this vital little part of the brain and its role in ADHD, brain-imaging studies have shown that the cerebellum is smaller in children and adults with ADHD,[4] and it is becoming clear that we should continue to explore its involvement in many more of the difficulties people with ADHD experience.

Connectivity – the brain's wiring

Our brains comprise areas or centres that can be described in terms of their function. We have a sound understanding of what many of these different areas do, based on studies of people who have lesions in well-defined parts of the brain due to injury or disease.

Even though there are large brain-imaging studies showing that certain brain areas are different in individuals with ADHD,[5] the problems experienced in ADHD are so complex that they can't simply be explained by these morphological variations in size.

The advances made in neuro-imagery in recent years have taught us that the neuronal connections *between* different areas of the brain can help explain many of the nuances of important human behaviour and function.[6] The current conception is that the brain's support tissue – myelin or 'white matter' – matures or develops later in ADHD. Consequently, the neurons' outgrowth, or axons, are less insulated and the nerve signals transmit less efficiently. This could explain some ADHD impairments as well as why it can manifest so differently from one individual to the next.

Think of this delay in maturation and its consequences as you would the lighting in a house, with the bulbs and light switches as the different brain areas, and the neuronal connections, axons, between them as the wiring. When the wires are poorly insulated or cut, the lights will flicker or go out, even if the bulbs and the switches are fully functional.

Dopamine – a key player

If I had a penny for every time someone with ADHD described to me how hard they find it to read a book, watch an entire film, or hold a conversation, I would be rich today. Imagine how difficult it would be to be constantly distracted by surroundings or internal thoughts. Not to mention how tiring a normal day in school or at work could be, triggering an emotional meltdown because of external stimuli others can filter out. These problems of regulating attention and emotions are closely associated with the neurotransmitter dopamine.

Clusters of neurons in various areas of the brain communicate with each other by releasing different neurotransmitters and activating electrical impulses that are spread through a highly complex network of axons (transmitters) and dendrites (receivers). Dopamine helps control many of our everyday behaviours as well as some of the more problematic ones. With the release of dopamine, we experience feelings of energy and pleasure. Very simply put, things that increase our chances of survival trigger the release of dopamine. By associating the dopamine-induced pleasure we experience with an event or behaviour, we learn to prioritize these events and behaviours over others. Dopamine helps the brain to evaluate, prioritize, and choose the activity that we need to act on in any given situation. With a dysregulated dopamine system, as with ADHD, it becomes harder to select the appropriate behaviour or activity among the myriad of stimuli with which our brains are constantly bombarded. Unfortunately, dopamine is also involved in the learning and choosing of things that, in the long run, are less beneficial for us, such as the consumption of addictive substances like nicotine, alcohol, and illicit drugs – substances that quickly and effectively release enormous amounts of dopamine.

The dopamine system thus also plays a role in why those with ADHD can find it so difficult to stop doing things perceived as rewarding and enjoyable. It can feel almost impossible to shift focus or activity once engaged in an activity – also referred to as hyperfocus.

Through brain imagery studies, we understand that the ADHD brain has problems with dopamine regulation.[7] There is either a surfeit or a dearth of the substance. If you have ADHD, it is harder to adapt energy levels, become motivated, and stay motivated to accomplish tasks.

For those with ADHD, all incoming information receives the same dopamine 'value'. Focus is jeopardized by new or different information. Much of our knowledge about ADHD comes from insights into the effects of a particular group of drugs on the core symptoms of the disorder. In the 1930s, US researchers discovered, by chance, that a group of amphetamine-based drugs – central stimulant agents – improved many of the ADHD symptoms. What began as an experiment to alleviate headaches in children with different forms of neurological disorders, proved instead to have beneficial effects on their hyperactivity, social skills, and academic performances.[8]

Cognition and consciousness – how we relate to ourselves and others

Much of what is going on in the brain and the theory behind different brain functions becomes difficult to understand due to the complicated language and technical terms used by psychiatrists and psychologists. In addition, not all expressions have a straightforward translation. Cognition and consciousness are terms commonly used but not always fully understood. This may be because they partially overlap. Cognition can be translated into 'knowing' and often implies a broader sense than just what we are consciously aware of. In a sense, everything encoded in our long-term memory is stuff that we 'know', even when we are not consciously accessing it. Conversely, consciousness is more than cognition since there are things that we experience without knowing exactly what they represent to us, such as some feelings and emotions. Thus, this becomes really messy as there are forms of cognition (i.e. knowing) that do not involve consciousness and there are forms of consciousness that do not involve cognition. For this purpose, and for the scope of this book, it will suffice to say that our consciousness and cognition will be the overarching terms under which some brain processes important to understand the underlying presentation of ADHD fit in.

Executive functions – the brain's flight control tower

Many people with ADHD can describe the feelings of frustration and sinking self-esteem that accompany the failure to complete everyday tasks that they know they can or should achieve. For many with ADHD, it becomes incredibly difficult to plan, organize, prioritize, and begin tasks that they know they need to tackle.

Both children and adults affected by ADHD also often find it harder than others to keep things in their memory, take decisions based on the best possible information, and adapt their behaviour to changing circumstances – or to the consequences of previous decisions or events that they have experienced.

To further complicate things, many with ADHD may be

extremely gifted in other areas and, for example, have strong verbal or social skills. ADHD may thus manifest differently in various people because of these unevenly distributed capacities, rendering a diagnosis difficult to understand and accept, both for those affected and for the people around them.

To better understand and grasp these complicated processes, we may compare our executive functions to the flight control tower at a large international airport. Our executive functions, much like the staff working in the control tower, will keep track of the myriad signals that the brain is exposed to at any given moment. This of course goes for both intrinsic (emotions and sensations from the body and all its organs) and extrinsic (stimuli from our complex surroundings) stimuli hitting our brain with sometimes contradictory signals. If the control tower is understaffed, as described by F in Chapter 9, all the incoming information quickly becomes overwhelming and unmanageable.

It is important to remember that the ADHD brain's control tower is not flawed or defective, but alternative. Usually, these impairments have very little to do with intelligence. In this sense, ADHD is not about knowing what has to be done; it's about not being able to do what has to be done, despite knowing that you have to do it.

Over and above planning, organizing, and prioritizing, the brain's control tower also regulates salience and motivation. It regulates our attention and energy levels so that we will keep going and put in that extra effort when things get complicated, or when there are distracting motivations. We need to be able to shift focus temporarily and then return to the task at hand. A good example of how important it is to be able to shift attention is when we are driving a car. When on the road, it's no help being hyperfocused on a particular object. To drive safely and efficiently, we need to be able to switch our focus and attention instantaneously. We need to assess and factor in multiple scenarios while constantly shifting our attention back to the road and the perpetually changing traffic situation. Many people with ADHD have difficulties in this respect, and indeed traffic accidents can be a serious consequence of the impaired executive functions and defects in complex attention in ADHD.

Another example would be complex, multi-step tasks. Multitasking is demanding for all brains. However, many adults with ADHD think of themselves as real pros when it comes to doing a lot of things simultaneously. The truth, however, is more often that multitasking results in energy loss due to problems in prioritizing and finishing tasks, managing a working day efficiently, or remembering items. Our executive functions also help us to activate the short-term working memory and retrieve experiences important to specific situations. It's also often difficult to remember and act on given instructions – in the proper order –to complete tasks and assignments.

In addition, the brain's control tower is responsible for gathering and handling time estimates for how long different things will take relative to each other. Besides having problems with memory retention, many with ADHD will tell us that they have a hard time learning and automating everyday tasks. Many will say that they feel forgetful and muddled, and that they often walk into a room and forget what they came in for. Some experience huge difficulties in school when learning vocabulary, multiplication tables, or schedules. It's common to hear adults with ADHD claiming to have no childhood memories, or that they find it hard to estimate how long ago something actually happened.

Our ability to express ourselves, to find the right words for a situation, or to coordinate body language and the intensity and pace of verbal communication also involves executive functions. We need to be able to talk about and describe experiences coherently and comprehensibly to others and to process and understand what others say and describe. For some people with ADHD, this is a serious problem; others are linguistically gifted and use their verbal faculties to compensate for impairments in other cognitive domains.

Perception, sensory input, and motor control
Perhaps you are one of those people with ADHD who is sensitive to impressions and sensory input from the outside world or signals from your own body? Many women with ADHD feel as if they lack a filter towards their surroundings and notice things that others do not register. Many with ADHD tell us they just can't stand the feel of their clothes against their body or that all the buzz of social situations exhausts them.

Although not included in the diagnostic criteria for ADHD, sensitivity to perceptual stimuli is more the rule than the exception in ADHD. Many people with ADHD will exhibit impairments in perception (sensory) and motor skills. Perception can be described as how our different senses receive, perceive, and react to external and internal stimuli or how we process visual and auditory information and coordinate these impressions with our voluntary movements. If these parts of the control tower's executive functions are affected, you may experience clumsiness or awkwardness. Someone may have had unreadable handwriting since childhood, another cannot catch a ball, while another is sensitive to smells or touch. Some might also find it hard to navigate familiar and unfamiliar environments – what is commonly referred to as our sense of direction.

Self-monitoring and self-perception

Something that rarely gets discussed in relation to ADHD is the social difficulty that impaired executive functions can cause. It is not always appreciated how important the brain's control tower is for self-monitoring, self-reflection, and self-control, which is to say how aware we are of our actions and behaviour. This also goes for our ability to handle frustration and to control our immediate emotions and impulses. Many adults with ADHD feel deeply ashamed about how they repeatedly upset their friends by blurting out something inappropriate or being unable to curb their language when angry. And we don't always get a second chance when we have said something to offend someone, no matter how sorry we are afterwards.

So, how is it all connected?

We can understand many of the problems and suffering associated with ADHD in terms of how different brain areas process information and communicate with each other. All the stimuli we receive from our external world need to be evaluated and prioritized through multiple brain networks for us to be able to choose a suitable behavioural response matching the most important information and the long- or short-term goals we wish to achieve. The brain's control tower works ceaselessly to create order from this chaos of incoming and outgoing signals.

Having ADHD is described by some as having a brain without a filter. Imagine your brain as a computer that suddenly loses the ability to sift out viruses and spam. You would be under constant attack. How would you sort it all out? What files would be safe to open and which email would you reply to first? What can wait?

The communication between the frontal lobes and other brain areas enables us to have a sense of time, to prioritize information, to structure our lives, and to resist immediate temptation in order to obtain deferred gratification. In ADHD, this communication, to different degrees, may be impaired. It may be displayed in everyday life as forgetting to bring things to work, not paying bills on time, or a hesitation to complete or sign off on tasks or assignments due to uncertainty.

This interconnectedness between the frontal lobes and the rest of the brain is not synonymous with intelligence. A person might be considered gifted and quick-witted yet she cannot get the agreed task done, the report written, or her part of the joint project handed in. If you don't understand that the intellect is not the same as executive function, but instead they are two disparate but parallel processes, it would be easy to place quick judgement on someone as either being lazy or manipulative.

However, it is important to remember that these difficulties are just as frustrating to understand for the person who has them as for others. When our executive functions are impaired, or put differently, when we are understaffed in the brain control tower, all information must be dealt with manually. Living with ADHD does not allow the luxury of an autopilot or using the brain's energy-saving functions as others might. Ostensibly well-meant advice to relax can therefore come across as hurtful and may also be counterproductive. With ADHD, maintaining control seems necessary to keep inner chaos in a constant state of order.

A famous psychological experiment called the 'Marshmallow Test' reveals that even by the age of four, children exhibit differences in self-control and their ability to delay immediate gratification in the hope of later reward.[9] Follow-up studies on the children who participated in these experiments also show that those who were able to control their impulses at an early age performed better at school later in life.[10]

We know today that in children with ADHD, there may be a lag of several years in the maturation of the frontal lobes, leaving them less able to control many important brain functions than their peers.[11] Again, delayed maturity in the frontal lobes has very little to do with intelligence or other talents, but clearly affects the brain's executive functions, making it more difficult to resist sudden impulses – such as telling your boss *exactly* what you feel about her management style, or eating the entire chocolate bar despite knowing it will make you sick. Living with ADHD often involves making hasty and impulsive decisions based on insufficient information and limited consequence analysis, which can give the impression that you don't understand what's best for you. However, as we now know, that is usually not the case.

S AND THE BROKEN SERVO

S, a young woman, described what it's like to live with impaired executive functions in a way that corresponds very well to the scientific understanding of ADHD. In a structured interview as part of her neuropsychological assessment for ADHD diagnostic criteria, S said:

'Yeah, all of those examples that you suggest fit. But it's more like I can never do anything in moderation. It's all or nothing for me, as if the servo in my volume control doesn't work properly.'

She continued: 'It's not that I don't know what to do; it's just that it doesn't get done.'

As a girl, S was often told that she was a real tomboy. She was active and outgoing and often hung around with her older brothers and their friends. S had a hot temper and would throw herself wholeheartedly into whatever activity she was engaged in. She believes she got away with her irascible temperament and emotional outbursts largely because she socialized almost exclusively with older boys.

'I guess they'd just find it funny and a bit cute when I'd explode after missing a penalty shot,' she said.

According to S's mother, S was a messy child. She would spread her things all over the house and her room looked like a perpetual war zone. S remembered that as a young girl she was self-confident, carefree, and largely unbothered by the mayhem she left in her wake. But as she grew older, she became more and more frustrated with her difficulties in organizing and creating order. Even though she would often start off cleaning, everything ended up a mess.

In her teens, things became even more tumultuous, not least emotionally. Her family and friends no longer found her outbursts innocently charming, and S felt ashamed, unable to regulate her emotional register. She was tossed from highest to lowest volume without being able to understand how to turn down her activity, energy, and emotions. Yet, some days, she couldn't even get the volume up at all.

'These days it feels as if I'm dead on the inside, like there's no point doing anything. The smallest demand feels overwhelming. Even though I know that on another day I'd have been able to do these things without a second thought. Things I enjoy, good things, also become problematic when my volume control goes up and I can't stop. Other people find me manic and think it strange that I can't just drop things. When I have all this energy, I start so many things at once that I lose all control of what needs to be done.

'It all turns into one big mess, and I end up finishing nothing. The hardest part is that I don't know when my energy is going to turn up or down. It can change so fast and for seemingly no logical reason and I end up letting people down.'

The difficulties S had planning, regulating, and controlling her energy levels, actions, emotions, and behaviour created problems in her life even though she knew what she should do and how she should do it. She felt as if she had no command over her inner volume control and as the years passed, this gnawed away at her self-esteem and self-image to the extent that she often felt despair and hopelessness.

Notes

1   Heide *et al.*, 2018
2   Gogtay *et al.*, 2004
3   Miquel *et al.*, 2019
4   Hoogman *et al.*, 2017
5   Hoogman *et al.*, 2017
6   Castellanos *et al.*, 2002
7   Del Campo *et al.*, 2011
8   Doyle, 2004
9   Mischel *et al.*, 1972
10   Mischel *et al.*, 1989
11   Hoogman *et al.*, 2017

Chapter 3

The Hormones

It shouldn't come as a huge surprise that some of the human population undergoes major hormonal changes several times every year. Female sex hormones not only fluctuate over months, but also over the entire lifespan, from puberty to menopause. However, since (until fairly recently) almost all research on ADHD was based on boys and men, the assessments of, and medications used for, ADHD are therefore primarily tested and tailored for a brain with a much more stable hormonal environment.

With the exception of how drug doses may be adjusted to the growing child, there has never been any serious discussion or research on how ADHD symptoms can change throughout different life phases or hormonal cycles for women, and that their medication may be affected by these quite extreme hormonal fluctuations. This is quite remarkable, given all the girls and women with ADHD who tell us how they lose control of their emotions and energy levels as they pass through puberty, during certain phases of their menstrual cycles, and during and after pregnancy. Older women with ADHD describe how their ADHD symptoms changed or worsened during menopause; that they suffer even more from brain fog, insomnia, and emotional dysregulation for many years around menopause. In periods of fluctuating hormones, many women, with and without ADHD, will experience debilitating cognitive difficulties, feel more impulsive and generally less able to function in their everyday lives.

Even if the research can provide few reliable explanations for how all this is related, we still need to take these testimonies seriously. More specifically, individual experiences in relation to hormonal factors must be accounted for when planning ADHD treatment and other interventions. Regrettably, this is not the case today. So, let's take a closer look at what happens in the female body and brain across the hormonal journey and how it might influence and affect ADHD.

A AND THE REOCCURRING AGGRESSIONS

A was diagnosed with ADHD while still at secondary school. It was highly unusual for girls to be diagnosed with ADHD at that time, but A presented with many of the symptoms of hyperactivity and impulsivity that are more common among boys.

It took many years before A started to connect the dots and detect a disturbing pattern in her intimate relationships. After she'd had yet another failed attempt at finding love, a friend suggested she download a 'period app'. A pattern of recurring periods of especially low self-esteem and melancholy, hypersensitivity, repulsion towards physical closeness, irritability, and, above all, a hair-trigger aggressivity, appeared every one or two weeks before she was due to menstruate.

In hindsight, A could easily identify several relationships that ended during these periods of negative affects – arguments that she bitterly regretted and friendships she was unable to save and subsequently grieved over for a long time afterwards. These problems have not become easier over the years; on the contrary, in fact. When she was in her twenties, these episodes of uncontrolled emotions and aggression would last for a couple of days before her period. Now, in her forties, it's more like a fortnight or more – over half the month, or half her life.

A thinks of the fortnight before her period as a time of 'ADHD deluxe', when her ADHD symptoms are amplified and defence mechanisms and otherwise well-rehearsed strategies prove to be ineffective. Today, A has control over much of these problems by keeping track of her cycles using a period app and tailoring her ADHD medications together with her psychiatrist. Much like someone with diabetes titrating insulin doses with respect to multiple externally and internally changing factors, she adjusts her doses to the different phases of her menstrual cycle and has greatly improved her emotion and anger management by this simple measure.

Also, the insight that her mental state can be attributed to biology has restored some of her damaged self-esteem. Planning ahead and being aware of her biological states helps her not to panic and make hasty decisions with unwanted long-term consequences during her more vulnerable periods.

Female hormones and the brain

ADHD symptoms will never exist in a vacuum but must be put in the context of the internal and external environment of the individual body and mind. This fact may be particularly true for women, since the female sex hormone oestrogen affects both the development and everyday function of the brain. Furthermore, a woman's hormone levels will vary greatly throughout life and during each menstrual cycle, affecting not only the reproductive organs but also the input and output of brain processes.

Unfortunately, too few studies have been conducted on how normal hormonal fluctuations affect ADHD symptoms in females. Even less is known about how endogenous hormones might interact with the different medications used to treat ADHD. But girls and women with ADHD keep telling us that their hormones matter. Until we have more concrete facts about this, there are some compelling theories that may help us deepen our understanding when assessing, diagnosing, and treating girls and women with ADHD.

On a theoretical level, animal studies show that oestrogen and dopamine are closely intertwined and mediate each other's effects. Oestrogen targets dopamine cells in the brain and stimulates enzymes involved in dopamine synthesis.[1] In addition, natural fluctuations of oestrogen and progesterone (another female sex hormone) during the menstrual cycle affect many of the cognitive processes in decision-making, social skills, and emotional regulation for women in general.[2] Even though there is still a lack of studies on how women with ADHD respond to hormonal fluctuations, there are several reports on how progesterone (natural as well as synthetic progestogens in contraceptives) affects women's moods.[3]

Furthermore, perhaps due to the interaction between oestrogen and dopamine, the effects of central stimulant drugs used to treat ADHD also seem to be affected by changes in sex hormones. Many women report that the effect of their medication is enhanced in the first part of the menstrual cycle (the follicular phase). During the first two weeks of the menstrual cycle, oestrogen levels rise while progesterone levels remain low. In the two latter weeks of the cycle (the luteal phase), progesterone levels rise, dampening the effect of the oestrogen.[4] Unfortunately, there are no studies exploring how hormonal fluctuations affect treatment or whether doses should be adjusted according to the menstrual cycle. Another interesting, yet unexplored hypothesis is whether contraceptives that even out hormone levels during the menstrual cycle could improve ADHD symptoms and emotional regulation in fertile women.

So, while there are many interesting and promising hypotheses, there is still a huge knowledge gap concerning how natural and synthetic hormonal fluctuations may alter, improve, or sometimes exacerbate underlying ADHD symptoms. A charitable explanation as to why so little research has been done on female ADHD symptoms in relation to hormonal fluctuations could be that these conditions are handled by different medical specialities. Gynaecologists specialize in female sex hormones, while ADHD and psychiatric comorbidities are handled by psychiatrists. So even though many women testify to a worsening of their ADHD symptoms and impaired everyday functionality in relation to certain periods of their menstrual cycle and hormonal changes across life, there is really very little hard evidence to guide us when we aim to alleviate distress and suffering associated with ADHD and hormones in girls and women.

Childhood

Ovaries, responsible for producing the female sex hormone are dormant from birth and do not do much during childhood. Stable hormonal levels combined with more subtle ADHD symptoms can make it difficult for others to understand and see the uphill struggle of girls during this phase of life. The chances of detecting ADHD in girls has improved since the diagnostic criteria for the age at which symptoms should manifest was raised from seven to 12. However, this age barrier for diagnosis remains problematic for females as many girls don't show externalizing symptoms before hormones kick in. For most, that will happen around or even after the age of 12.

As puberty approaches, the ovaries start producing oestrogen at an increasing rate until the first ovulation occurs. From that point on, oestrogen and progesterone are produced and synchronized effectively every month in a regular cycle.

Puberty, adolescence, and reproductive health

The teenage years are a time of both possibilities and challenges. For many, the years around puberty and into adolescence can be turbulent and frightening. That goes both for teenagers and their parents.

Consequently, teenage years create friction and conflict in many families, causing many parents to ask what on earth could be the point of all the tears and shouting. As a parent of five teenagers, I'm more than aware of this, and, to be quite honest, cannot look back at my own teenage years with any unmitigated pride either. I probably got back exactly what I deserved. However, when the teenage tsunami hits, I often find it helpful and comforting to take a step back and think about the evolutionary benefits for creating such strife within an often well-knit group of genetically related individuals.

But the truth is that our species depends on teenagers

questioning their parents, as this friction will set them off on a (often quite hazardous) journey towards becoming autonomous individuals. If we just stayed home with our parents, there would be no new children made, and nature can't have that. Interestingly enough, evolution has made sure that our brains – especially the frontal lobes – remain undeveloped during this period of life. Somehow it seems as if nature wants us to take all these risks and to prioritize our friends' norms over our parents' advice – probably since it is important for the survival of our species that we are accepted by our peers and form new social groups that can lead to forming our own families.

Unfortunately, adolescence and the radical changes that the body and brain undergo can also be associated with a higher risk of stress, social insecurity, and mental ill-health. This appears to be particularly true for adolescent girls and women with ADHD. One US study that followed girls and young women with ADHD from childhood into adulthood shows that women with ADHD describe their teenage years as especially challenging. They struggle both academically and socially at school, start smoking, drinking, and taking drugs earlier and suffer from depression and anxiety more often than girls without a diagnosis. Unfortunately, it's common that it is not until they reach their teens or young adulthood that their problems become obvious to others.[5]

Furthermore, girls and young women with ADHD frequently suffer from low self-esteem and peer rejection, often ending up in risky situations. This is particularly true when it comes to relationships and sex. Research shows that girls and women with ADHD have sex at an earlier age and with more partners than their same-aged peers. Due to a vicious spiral catalyzed by a longing for love and approval, they are at risk for all kinds of negative reproductive health outcomes, such as sexually transmitted diseases, unplanned pregnancies, abortions, and early unintentional parenthood.[6] In fact, our research group recently showed that girls and women with ADHD have a sixfold increased risk of becoming teenage mothers compared to young women without a diagnosis.[7]

It is not yet known exactly why women with ADHD are at elevated risk of becoming teenage mothers. Core symptoms of ADHD, such as impaired cognitive function, executive dysfunction, and impulsivity, will inevitably play in to the risk of becoming a teenage mother. ADHD can make it difficult to remember to take your oral contraceptives, and common comorbidities and psychosocial consequences of low self-esteem and peer rejection can put young females with ADHD in situations where it's difficult to 'stand your ground'. Many young women with ADHD tell us that they have agreed to sexual situations that they in fact were not at all comfortable with. Mental and emotional side-effects of contraceptives are relatively prevalent among young women and especially common in women with previous mental health issues. Indeed, many young women with ADHD will tell us that they stopped taking the pill due to side-effects and try to use other, perhaps less effective, methods.[8]

In another recent study from our research group, we found that young women with ADHD had more problems tolerating hormonal contraceptives compared to their unaffected peers. More specifically, they had a fivefold increased risk of developing depression following oral contraceptive use compared to unaffected women of the same age.[9] Since parenthood in early age overlaps with important and formative years in life, this risk enhances the negative psychosocial outcomes already associated with ADHD. Thus, since the contraceptive methods selected should not confer unnecessary risks of mood dysregulation and depression, effective alternatives must be easily available to them. User-independent, long-acting, reversible contraception such as intrauterine devices (IUDs) may be a safe and effective way of preventing teenage pregnancies in young women with ADHD.

Unfortunately, since women with psychiatric diagnoses are often excluded from scientific studies of contraceptives, we still know too little about this pressing issue. More research on women's unique biological conditions and ADHD would likely dramatically improve the quality of life for girls and women affected by ADHD.

The menstrual cycle

Most girls have their first period between the age of ten and 16. The average menstrual cycle lasts about 28 days but can vary by up to four days before being considered irregular. Ovulation normally occurs 14 days prior to the menstrual bleeding.

Assuming a 28-day menstrual cycle, oestrogen levels will gradually rise during the first two weeks of the follicular phase. No progesterone is produced during this time, and the oestrogen will stimulate the release of other important brain neurotransmitters such as serotonin and dopamine. Previous research shows that oestrogen positively affects executive function and attention in women in general.[10] We know less about how hormonal fluctuations affect ADHD symptoms in girls and women, but it comes as no great surprise to hear that many women with ADHD find the first two weeks following menstruation less problematic, both emotionally and in terms of everyday functioning.

On a higher level, in the brain, two overarching hormones,

secreted from the pituitary gland – follicle stimulating hormone (FSH) and luteinizing hormone (LH) – stimulate the ovaries to produce oestrogen and trigger ovulation. After ovulation, around day 14, the follicle (or egg sac) turns into the hormone-producing corpus luteum (yellow body). The corpus luteum secretes progesterone, which prepares the uterine lining (endometrium) for the arrival of a fertilized egg and a potential following pregnancy. So, during the last two weeks of the menstrual cycle, the luteal phase, progesterone levels rise along with the already high and stable oestrogen levels. There is some indication that progesterone has the potential to aggravate ADHD-like symptoms, and women with ADHD correspondingly often report that the luteal phase is associated with worsening of their ADHD symptoms and everyday functioning.[11]

PMS or PMDD

Many women describe themselves as being especially delicate and unstable with sudden and intrusive mood swings, anxiety, irritability, and sleep disruption days or weeks before their periods. PMS (premenstrual syndrome) and PMDS (premenstrual dysphoric disorder), a more debilitating form of PMS, are conditions that often cause impairing psychological and physical symptoms. Research shows that PMS and PMDS are more common in women with ADHD than in the general population.[12]

Accounts of how common it is for fertile women to experience PMS- or PMDD-related problems differ. This is largely due to how the symptoms are defined and at what point they are considered problematic. Furthermore, we don't know exactly what causes PMS or PMDD and why some women suffer more than others. However, there are numerous theories of what happens in the body when oestrogen and progesterone levels fluctuate over a menstrual cycle. Although it has not been fully explored, oestrogen is sometimes considered to be a 'super fuel' for the brain, enhancing cognitive and executive functions, improving sleep quality, memory, and emotional regulation. Oestrogen appears to have a protective effect for women's overall mental health throughout life. In contrast, on a theoretical level, PMS and PMDD symptoms are thought to be linked to rising levels of progesterone during the luteal phase, and there are some indications that progesterone, or metabolites of progesterone, may have a detrimental effect on some women and their ability to handle anxiety and feelings of aggression. Thus, progesterone has the potential to worsen ADHD control and everyday functioning.[13]

Handling ADHD is often tough enough as it is, but on top of this many girls and women must manage their ADHD during constant hormonal fluctuation. A core ingredient for successful ADHD management is self-insight and self-awareness. It is not hard to understand that this may be many times harder to achieve if everything, including hormones, emotions, and ADHD symptoms, is constantly changing. We need to draw attention to these difficulties and provide the right support to mitigate the risk of impaired ADHD symptoms due to PMS and PMDS in both the short and long term.

Pregnancy

Many women, with or without ADHD, will become mothers at some point in their lives. However, not all of them will be prepared for how this 'natural state of exception' will impact their hormonal balance and mental well-being. The growing placenta produces hormones that affect many of the body's organs, including hormone release from the adrenal and thyroid glands that can affect the central nervous system and the brain.

There is today no way to predict how any one woman will react physically or emotionally to these hormone changes. That said, with different hormone levels changing over a short period of time, many women experience tiredness and mood swings during the first few months of pregnancy, whether or not they have ADHD.

When oestrogen increases during pregnancy, many women can tell that they feel and function better – again regardless of their ADHD status. However, if a woman's ADHD is associated with impaired body image, her ability to cope with change, or her sensitivity to hormonal fluctuations, the pregnancy can prove more difficult.

Pregnant women with ADHD commonly report feelings of being uncomfortable in their growing body, worry about the uncertainties of labour and their ability to cope with pain, or are plagued by self-doubt in the face of imminent motherhood. Often, the understanding of one's ADHD symptoms and the accompanying support from others proves crucial to determine the outcome of a woman's pregnancy. Many women choose to discontinue their ADHD medication ahead of or during pregnancy in the belief that too little is still known about if and how these drugs might affect them and their foetus.

Until recently, there was simply not enough research data from women using ADHD medication during pregnancy to give clear and general advice. However, today we don't have any evidence that central stimulant medication will harm the pregnant mother or her unborn child. In practice, as with most pharmacological treatments during pregnancy, it often becomes a transparent risk versus benefit discussion with the woman and her partner. The choice to continue or suspend medication should always be based on the individual woman's preference, the level of ADHD symptoms, and potential consequences. A thorough examination by a psychiatrist and a gynaecologist with extensive experience in ADHD and obstetric risk factors, preferably working together, is always recommended. Some women will opt to suspend their treatment, while others decide to continue. Either way, what we know is that the most important thing for both mother and baby is to feel as mentally, emotionally, and functionally well during the pregnancy as possible.[14,]

Childbirth and early motherhood

To welcome a child into this world can be one of the most special and joyful moments in life. However, for some, this experience may also be perceived as both frightening and uncertain. It's not unusual for women to feel low or even depressed after pregnancy and childbirth. This may be particularly true for new parents with ADHD. In fact, research shows that postpartum depression is more common in women with ADHD, compared to the general population.[15] The shame and taboo that may accompany these forbidden emotions are often an extra burden in an already heavy situation. For some, what initially feels like a temporary mood dip can deteriorate into a state of out-and-out angst and depression in which they become mired in gloomy thoughts, paralysing fatigue, or feelings of fear and impending disaster.

Understanding the basics about living with ADHD makes it easy to see how childbirth and infancy can pose serious threats to the mental well-being of a new mother. For someone who is normally susceptible to insomnia, the first months with a demanding newborn can be an extra challenge. And for someone with difficulties organizing their own everyday life, the extra organizational skills and emotional stress tolerance needed to care for a baby with unpredictable claims on them and their body can feel quite impossible.

Even though there is still limited research on the risk of postnatal depression in women with ADHD, we do know that a serious and negative perinatal experience is a risk factor. Considering how ADHD leaves a person more susceptible to anxiety and depression and perceived difficulties in establishing routines and a functional structure in life, it's easy to understand how women can be extra sensitive when hormonal swings coincide with major life-changing events.

It's therefore essential that we are aware of, and, if possible, prevent, severe forms of stress and depression following pregnancy and childbirth. Much is gained if we can make a concrete plan ahead of delivery, together with the pregnant mother, her partner, family, and healthcare professionals. This plan should be as specific as possible and include the mother's expectations and fears, but also a detailed description of how she wants others to act and support her based on her underlying ADHD and/or other unique vulnerabilities. The aim should always be to give her and the child the best possible start in their new life together.

Menopause and ageing

Along with the realization that ADHD is not just a diagnosis concerning children and young adults, we have come to realize that a substantial number of adult women will enter yet another period in life that may be specially challenging for those with ADHD. Menopause, which for most women will occur at around the age of 50, represents the end of her fertile years where oestrogen levels will gradually decrease until no more endogenous hormone is produced. Menopause is defined as one year (12 months) after a woman's last period. The mean age for this is 51 years.

However, this gradual decline in oestrogen generally starts about five to ten years before the actual menopause. With a mean age of about 47, most woman enter a period called perimenopause when periods become more irregular and occur in both longer and shorter intervals. The menstruation can be heavy in some periods and light in others. This is due to increasingly irregular, but over time gradually decreasing, levels of oestrogen and progesterone. The levels of the two overarching hormones, FSH and LH, stimulating the ovaries to produce oestrogen and to release the egg, will also fluctuate considerably during perimenopause. Initially, FSH and LH will increase as a response to decreasing oestrogen levels, but over time they will also decrease and remain low entering menopause. Thus, FSH and LH can be used to assess a woman's stage of peri- or post-menopause.

Entering menopause, ovulation ceases, thus no progesterone is produced either, and for some women symptoms of PMS/ PMDS can wane and eventually disappear. However, these fluctuating hormone levels during peri- and menopause may also be associated with more extreme mood dysregulation and cognitive impairments for many women, ADHD or not.[16]

For women with ADHD, this period of life can be particularly distressing and disabling. Just as fluctuating oestrogen levels affect the body and brain during the monthly menstrual cycles, the increased and irregular fluctuation across perimenopause and the depleted oestrogen levels following menopause will impact the brain in many ways.

For some women, these internal changes, together with new life circumstances (perhaps retirement, relocation, or losing friends, loved ones, or even a life partner) become more stressful than for others. The decline in oestrogen also affects levels of serotonin and dopamine, further affecting mood, emotional regulation, memory, energy levels, and stress tolerance. Many women with ADHD report that their pre-existing symptoms worsen in the years surrounding menopause. Some describe the onset of ADHD symptoms that they have never experienced before.

A subset of women with or without an ADHD diagnosis will experience severe memory impairments and will seek medical help, concerned that they might be developing dementia or Alzheimer's disease. In the case of not previously having been diagnosed with ADHD, this can pose quite a challenge during the assessment, trying to disentangle what symptoms are best attributed to what condition: ADHD, dementia, or menopause?

For women with an existing ADHD diagnosis entering menopause, it is not uncommon to find that their hormonal changes affect both ADHD medication and previous successful coping strategies. Sometimes patients and their doctors must readdress the condition to discover new ways forward.

Sexuality and relationships

Sexuality is a private and, for many people, sensitive matter. Unfortunately, questions about this important aspect of life are rarely addressed in ADHD assessment and treatment. Could this be because it's considered an especially private and sensitive matter for women in general? Or because there is no real research that has explored whether, and if so how, women with ADHD experience specific challenges when it comes to their sexuality and intimate relationships?

We do, however, have reason to believe that the impairments associated with ADHD also impact this private sphere of our lives. After all, many of the problems experienced by people with ADHD can be traced back to the dysregulation of crucial brain functions, and many women with the diagnosis describe how they occasionally have difficulties linked to their sexuality, libido, and ability to derive pleasure from sex.

Perhaps you are just so totally exhausted by your efforts to hold your life together that the very idea of having sex feels like yet another obstacle? Or maybe is it that nagging restlessness and the need for novelty that makes it impossible for you to stay with one partner?

The brain's reward system, steering our behaviour towards increased chance of survival, is very much engaged in the sexual act. The brain has therefore made sure to reward us with a veritable deluge of dopamine when we have sex. Given that we also know that ADHD is associated with difficulties regulating dopamine levels, and that those with ADHD are more inclined to have problems with behaviours involving motivation and reward, it is not a surprise that sex also can become problematic. Consequently, this vulnerability applies to gambling, alcohol, food, and drugs as well as sex.

In addition, the impulsivity that is one of the core features of ADHD can also be a hindrance when it comes to sex and relationships. It's seldom a particularly good idea to act on a sudden sexual impulse if you're already in a highly valued monogamous relationship – at least if you hope to nurture and sustain it and genuinely share your partner's values and belief that exclusive sex is non-negotiable.

However, with the right explanatory model, support, and self-awareness, it is possible to lead a full and rich life with ADHD despite a reward system wired slightly differently.

Notes

1   Kuppers *et al.*, 2000
2   Dreher *et al.*, 2007
3   Sundström Poromma *et al.*, 2020
4   Justice & de Wit, 1999, 2000; White *et al.*, 2002
5   Hinshaw *et al.*, 2012
6   Barkley, 2006; Østergaard *et al.*, 2017
7   Skoglund *et al.*, 2019
8   Bengtsdotter *et al.*, 2018
9   Lundin *et al.*, 2022
10 Hatta & Nagaya, 2009
11 Roberts *et al.*, 2018
12 Dorani *et al.*, 2021
13 Lundin *et al.*, 2022
14 Jiang *et al.*, 2019; Freeman, 2014; McAllister-Williams *et al.*, 2017
15 Dorani *et al.*, 2021
16 Weber *et al.*, 2013

Chapter 4

The Invisible Girls

As mentioned previously, ADHD has historically been a disorder more frequently diagnosed in boys. According to different studies, one girl is diagnosed with ADHD to every 3–16 boys, with this skewed distribution being more prominent in childhood and in clinical populations, levelling out in adulthood.[1]

There are several reasons for this gender asymmetry. As a group, girls are more often diagnosed with the inattentive form of ADHD, ADD.[2] In general, symptoms of inattention may be harder than those of hyperactivity and impulsivity to perceive and understand. Put simply, girls are more commonly diagnosed with the form of ADHD that doesn't disturb others. They lag behind and fail in peer relationships without causing trouble for anyone but themselves. Moreover, they tend to blame the consequences of these disappointments on themselves. Parents, schools, youth clinics, and healthcare services therefore often overlook them, illustrating a serious paradox in childhood ADHD – girls are diagnosed with ADHD less frequently, while being just as susceptible to its adverse consequences.[3]

It is not true that all boys and men with ADHD are overly active, oppositional, aggressive, and disturbing and that all girls and women with ADHD turn their struggles inwards. Girls and women can display many signs of hyperactivity and impulsivity if we know what to look for. But symptoms of hyperactivity and impulsivity in females, such as consequences of emotional dysregulation, self-harm, or sexual risk taking, are frequently attributed to other conditions (such as borderline personality disorder) or explained by social or environmental factors (such as adverse upbringing, negative peer influence, or trauma). Sadly, when girls exhibit symptoms of hyperactivity and impulsivity, it is often referred to as defiance and externalization. The same behaviours in boys, however, are more commonly interpreted as 'typical ADHD symptoms'.[4]

In studies when teachers were presented with hypothetical descriptions of children who display specific issues, they frequently recommended support, accommodations, and treatment for male names or pronouns. This was the same even when the vignettes used were identical except for the child's suggested sex.[5] Unfortunately, this gender bias towards noticing and attending to the boys also seems true for parents, who more often underestimate impairment and the severity of their daughters' hyperactive and impulsive symptoms as compared to their sons'.[6] Again, it seems like we have a tendency to attribute girls' problems to different types of traumatic life events, while boys' problematic behaviours are put down to medical or genetic factors. However, parents seem to do better at identifying a problem than teachers. Researchers speculate that this may be due to parents' tendency to compare their own daughters with same-aged girls, while teachers draw such comparisons with boys in the same class.[7]

Another reason that we miss girls with ADHD is that they

often present with psychiatric comorbidity in the form of internalizing disorders like anxiety, depression, obsessive-compulsive disorder (OCD), and compensatory strategies such as perfectionism, which tends to recommend other psychiatric diagnoses before ADHD. Girls and adolescent women with ADHD struggle with social, relational, and psychosexual problems. They often experience emotional instability and difficulties regulating energy levels that hinder the development of sustainable and healthy coping strategies. Indeed, their quality of life and self-esteem are often dramatically affected by problems in managing and maintaining peer relationships, making it harder for them to access positive social networks and peer support.[8]

Every year a girl spends without the proper diagnosis increases the risk of her developing more serious problems once she finally comes for assessment and treatment. Sadly, even once diagnosed with ADHD, girls receive less support and treatment compared to same-aged boys with the diagnosis. Indeed, research shows that boys are more likely to be given a psychiatric diagnosis as the explanation for their difficulties where the same symptoms in girls are more rarely deemed to meet the criteria of a diagnosis, the very prerequisite to receive treatment. Consequently, boys receive both medical treatment and counselling more often than girls.[9]

Thus, the barriers for detection and the delay of diagnosis in girls and women are still very much the reality. Thanks to dedicated researchers and clinicians, however, things are slowly changing, with important advances towards better understanding of the unique challenges for girls and women with ADHD.

Self-esteem and relationships

Humans are social creatures – to what degree, however, differs greatly between individuals. Most of us are born with innate and rudimentary social skills that will secure our immediate survival. We develop more advanced social competence gradually during childhood and fine tune it in adolescence and early adulthood. As we grow older, our social skills will become increasingly important to our development towards independent adults. We must manage more and more advanced things without the support of our caregivers and have to adapt to the demands of present and future circumstances. Mutual (successful) interaction with peers and adults helps us to acquire the self-esteem and self-image we need to be accepted by and co-exist with others.

Many girls and women with ADHD paint a gloomy picture of their quality of life and mental health.[10] They report feeling more different and are more ashamed of themselves and their problems than boys with ADHD, with more stress and loss of control in their lives than other girls their age.[11] These experiences of stress, low self-esteem, and social impediments follow the girls through their lives and impact their adult relationships.[12]

Sadly, research proves them right in feeling gloomy about their future. It turns out that girls' 'ADHD behaviour' is less tolerated and more often criticized by others than in boys. Indeed, many girls with ADHD report feeling increasingly alienated and different, not fitting in anywhere.[13]

Females with ADHD also find it harder to manage their social network and interpersonal relationships. They have fewer friendships, as they tend to end up in more volatile situations, arguments, and conflicts. Sadly, they are also less liked by adults and tend to be bullied and ostracized more than those without ADHD.[14] Not surprisingly, in light of this, girls with ADHD also often expect to be less well received by both adults and their peers than girls without ADHD.

Consequently, many girls and women with ADHD talk about perpetually sinking self-esteem, even self-contempt, stemming from feelings of not fitting in. Many desperately wish they could behave differently. Knowing what we know about the inherited difficulties in ADHD, it makes sense that the diagnosis may have negative consequences in relationships and academic and professional settings. Given that ADHD often makes it difficult to perceive and assimilate information at a sufficient speed, social situations can be extremely challenging.

Longitudinal and observational studies of girls with ADHD show that teenage girls with pronounced inattention are more likely to stay at home with their parents and remain friendless.[15] This is more than just unfair and sad. Additionally, it can be harmful, both in the present and future, to those who are excluded and unable to maintain friendships they long for.

O AND THE ACCEPTANCE OF BEING DIFFERENT

Many girls and women with ADHD describe feelings of belonging to a minority that this world wasn't made for. A colleague of mine told me about her now 17-year-old daughter, O.

O was diagnosed with ADD when she was 16, having struggled for many years both in school and with friendships. On and off throughout her life, she had battled with periods of anxiety and self-doubt, depression, and insomnia.

As a child, O was an unusually quiet and passive little girl, and her family grew worried. Her mother, my colleague, contacted a neurologist to ask if her daughter might have epilepsy with absence seizures. This can be diagnosed or ruled out via an electroencephalogram (EEG), a technique to register the brain's electrical activity via electrodes placed against the skull. A referral and a few months' wait later, it was time for the procedure. Her mother prepared little O carefully: 'They're going to place stickers and wires to your head and you'll have to sit really still, but it won't hurt. This will help us see if there's something wrong or something different about your brain.' O conducted herself in exemplary fashion.

A few weeks later, the results arrived in the post. EEG: No anomalies found. My colleague picked O up from preschool and in the car on the way home she said: 'Do you remember that time we stuck wires on your head to look at your brain? Everything was normal. Your brain is completely normal.'

She had thought that O wouldn't have had such vivid memories of the examination, especially not since the girl didn't seem to react or register much in her surroundings at all, so she wasn't prepared for her daughter's reaction: 'What? That can't be right!'

O, who nine difficult years later would be assessed for and diagnosed with ADHD, predominantly inattentive type (ADD), already knew by the age of five that something was different about her brain. The following quote from O, aged five years old is one of the earliest and purest descriptions I've heard of that illustrates the experience of living with ADHD and feeling different:

'No, I'm not like other people. But that's okay; I've known it all along. I'm different and I'm fine with it.'

The expectations

Are there unwritten social and cultural expectations of what it means to be female? Probably. Do these impact those living with ADHD? Most likely.

'I'm the smartest dumb person I know. I'm one of those messy purse girls.'[16]

The quote is from an adult woman with ADHD describing herself as the girl whose handbag ('purse' in US English) is always a total mess – a fact that by now should not come as a surprise. Bearing in mind that ADHD causes difficulties in organizing and structuring your life, we probably shouldn't expect a well-ordered handbag from a woman with ADHD. However, a more important question is attached to our assumption here: Do we subconsciously also assume that women with tidy handbags by default are more conscientious, intelligent, and competent? Is a clean and smart handbag an indirect sign of academic achievement, popularity, and personal integrity? How well do we know our prejudices, really? We might not want to admit it, but do we let a characteristic that we frown on colour how we perceive other, unrelated characteristics?

Whether we care to admit it or not, this is in fact often what we do. The phenomenon even has its own name, the Halo Effect. For many girls and women, living with ADHD brings about a perpetually flagging self-esteem that is hard to cope with. They struggle hard from an early age, trying to cover up the impairments they were born with, so that others don't draw unfavourable conclusions about them and their personality.

Many girls and women with ADHD say that they put a great deal of effort into hiding and compensating for their problems. They overcompensate and end up in patterns of extreme behaviour in order to fit in. This daily battle to conceal an inner turmoil can give rise to exaggerated perfectionism, anxiety, social anxiety, eating disorders, or harmful alcohol and drug use. Afraid of losing control over their emotions and energy levels, they rarely know any other way of functioning. Many devote endless time and attention to trying to function on a basic level.

When someone constantly struggles to keep a threatening inner chaos at arm's length, they might find it unbearably hard to let details remain unfinished or incomplete. Others often only see the dysfunctional coping strategies, the overly organized, the inflexible or the perfectionistic side of the matter. Failing to see that it is deficiencies that causes a girl to be so hard on herself and others, people often try to get her to relax and lower her standards. To live a little and not be such a 'good girl' all the time. Surely this is not the most appreciated advice for someone struggling to keep the most basic things together.

How do we find the girls in time?

To understand the special challenges facing girls with ADHD, we need to take into account the factors that can be tacit in girls and women, including natural fluctuations of hormones, reaction to trauma, family dynamics, self-esteem, cultural context, and social expectations. As described earlier, girls' ADHD symptoms seem to be harder for others to detect and interpret than boys. Part of the explanation for this is probably due to a tendency to lay a cultural and social filter over our interpretation of girls' and boys' behaviours and problems. But it often also depends on girls being resourceful at finding strategies for handling their impairments and that they tend, more than boys, to turn their emotions inward.

So, what do we need to know to be able to detect and diagnose girls and women with ADHD earlier and prevent years of struggles?

Other symptom manifestations

The inattentive form of ADHD (ADD) is more commonly diagnosed in girls. Females might be diagnosed later, but that doesn't mean they are invisible. They and their parents often seek help early, but look for help with other psychiatric conditions, such as anxiety, depression, self-harming behaviour, dependency, or eating disorders, rather than ADHD. Their ADHD symptoms will only be found if we can see beyond their comorbidities and ask informed questions to unmask the strategies they use to hide the consequences of hyperactivity, impulsivity, and inattention.

Comorbidity

Anxiety and depression are common reasons why females seek care and support. When evidence-based interventions, which are normally effective to relieve anxiety and depression, don't work, it is logical to then consider an underlying neurodevelopmental vulnerability such as ADHD.

In today's society, we ascribe considerable weight and status to appearance, physique, and performance. ADHD causes difficulties controlling and curbing behaviours that pose threats to achieving many of those desirable attributes. For example, having problems regulating your appetite will cause many girls to struggle with their weight and dietary habits from a young age. Some will turn to occasional binge-eating and self-starvation, while others restrict their diet in an anorectic way to avoid losing control.

The association between ADHD and different eating disorders is described in research literature, and tallies well with the testimonies of many females with ADHD.

Some girls with ADHD have experienced trauma or abuse in their life. The symptoms of trauma often overlap with those of ADHD and are not mutually exclusive. The complex and unfair truth is that girls and women are more prone to exposure to situations of risk-causing trauma specifically *because of* their ADHD. Furthermore, their very ADHD will make them more susceptible to adverse reactions to trauma, such as developing PTSD, following similar traumatic events as peers without ADHD. Nonetheless, many females with undiagnosed ADHD are presented with flawed interpretations of their symptoms as merely consequences of earlier traumatic events.

Gender role expectations
Whether we like it or not, different structural social expectations are placed on both genders. This informs how we interpret behaviour. Many seem more accepting of the reserved, bashful behaviour of girls, and more accepting of a rule-breaking son over a daughter with the same behaviour.

Social impairments associated with an externalizing expression of ADHD are more shameful for females than males. Society expects girls to be well mannered, compliant, unobtrusive, and subordinate to adults. In some literature, this is described as part of a 'feminine socialization'. It's easy to understand that if such 'femininity' is part of our social structures, it does not fit with ADHD symptoms of impulsivity, restlessness, impatience, low frustration tolerance, verbal impulsivity, and difficulties with punctuality and scholastic performance.

Perhaps the same externalizing behaviour is more compatible with the accepted notion of how boys conduct themselves under society's masculine norms. That same behaviour, when observed in females with ADHD, is seen as clumsy and raucous, and creates 'social violations' at school, at home, among friends, and at work.

ADHD often negatively affects the self-confidence and self-image of girls and women in relation to society's norms and values. Never truly fitting in can cause considerable suffering.

When other family members have ADHD
It is well established that ADHD is influenced by genetic factors and up to 80 per cent of the risk of being affected, for both sexes, is thought to be due to heritability.[17] Thus, if a family member is diagnosed with or has symptoms of ADHD, there is a higher risk that other family members also are affected, regardless of the sex of the individual and even if the symptoms manifest differently from male to female.

Conflicts and school absenteeism
We still have a tendency to attribute girls' struggles in school with psychosocial explanations. For boys with the same problems, we often look to ADHD first. Therefore, when girls

are unable to adjust to demands and expectations of school, we should consider ADHD.

Externalizing and risk-taking behaviours

Even though ADHD can be a silent disability in girls, many describe a pattern of dramatic and volatile relationships, particularly from their teenage years and onwards.

Families with daughters with ADHD describe frequent and energy-draining conflict at home, even though the girl can often pull herself together at school or with peers. As girls with ADHD grow up, they expose themselves to more risks than unaffected female peers. Many of them experiment early with sex and substances. Indeed, research shows that adolescent girls and young adult women with ADHD will engage in hazardous use of alcohol, illicit drugs, and sexual risk-taking at a significantly higher degree than same-aged females without ADHD.[18] As a consequence, they are at high risk for sexually transmitted diseases, unplanned pregnancies, and victimization.[19] Therefore, when we meet these risk-taking girls, we must look to ADHD.

Strong reactions to hormonal fluctuations

As described previously, female oestrogen levels vary greatly across the menstrual cycle, affecting many different brain processes and functions. Much is still unknown, but there is already research that supports the hypothesized interaction between oestrogen and dopamine, potentially affecting ADHD throughout the menstrual cycle.[20] Therefore, when females describe an exacerbation of negative consequences from emotional dysregulation or dysfunctional coping strategies associated with hormonal fluctuation (e.g. severe forms of PMS/PMDS), we should consider ADHD.

What happens to the girls we miss?

So what do we – or rather these girls, women, and their families – risk if we carry on overlooking their ADHD symptoms and impairments?

In the short term, both research and experience tell us what many ADHD girls and women and their loved ones have been saying for a long time. Namely that these girls, without the correct explanatory model and adequate accommodations, may struggle with future academic failure, wrecked relationships, mental and physical comorbidity, and low self-esteem. Unfortunately, the gloomy story seldom ends there and ADHD in childhood and adolescence casts a long, dark shadow over these girls' futures as well.[21]

The developing personality and self-image of girls will unconditionally be damaged by constant failure during childhood and adolescence. More specifically, women with ADHD continue to experience severe lifestyle-related stress throughout their lives as well as feelings of being unable to influence their situation.

Notes

1 Gershon, 2002
2 Mowlem et al., 2019b
3 Biederman et al., 1999; Gershon, 2002; Hinshaw et al., 2012
4 Young et al., 2020
5 Pisecco et al., 2001; Sciutto et al., 2004
6 Mowlem et al., 2019a
7 Ohan & Visser, 2009; Gardner et al., 2002
8 Biederman et al., 1999; Hinshaw, 2002; Mowlem et al., 2019b
9 Derks et al., 2007; Gardner et al., 2002
10 Thurber et al. 2002
11 Rucklidge et al. 2007; Rucklidge & Tannock 2001

12 Arcia & Conners 1998
13 Quinn & Wigal, 2004; Quinn, 2005
14 Kok *et al.*, 2016
15 Kopp, 2010; Quinn & Madhoo, 2014
16 Keltner & Taylor, 2002
17 Thapar *et al.*, 2013
18 Hosain *et al.*, 2012
19 Young *et al.*, 2020
20 Roberts *et al.*, 2018
21 Young *et al.*, 2020

Chapter 5

The Emotions

ADHD isn't a mental illness and people with ADHD live in and perceive reality in exactly the same way as anyone else. However, being unable to suppress an emotional outburst only to have to endure other people's – and your own – frustration and exhaustion minutes or hours later often creates a recurring vicious circle of eruptions and apologies.

Even if difficulties handling, regulating, and adapting emotions are not included in the diagnostic criteria for ADHD, it's a problem that has been described in the literature for decades. In fact, many girls and women with ADHD specifically tell us that their emotional dysregulation is one of the major problem-creators in their lives.

A chapter on emotions has its self-evident place in a book on ADHD beyond the diagnostic criteria – not only because emotions are vital to us, but also because they have long been *excluded* from the diagnostic criteria. This is very much at odds with the accounts of all the girls and women living with ADHD, who commonly say that it is these very difficulties that have caused them the greatest setbacks and sorrows in life.

An emotional roller-coaster is more the rule than the exception when living with ADHD. This is not unique for females with ADHD, but it's a common reason why girls and women seek help and treatment. As will be described in more detail in the next chapter on comorbidities, ADHD-induced emotional instability is not the same as bipolar disorder or borderline disorder (emotionally unstable personality disorder). The diagnoses can, however, overlap and co-exist with ADHD.

Many girls and women with ADHD say they would prefer to not feel any emotions at all over their internal emotional turbulence. In light of the suffering that comes with difficulty regulating emotions, this is easy to understand.

Our emotions are messengers of important information that, on the most primitive level, will help us make decisions to improve our chances of survival. We encounter an unknown danger, feel fear, and withdraw. We get threatened or attacked, feel anger, and defend ourselves. We see something exciting and new, feel curiosity, and approach it. We smell rotten food, feel disgusted, and reject it. And so on.

But our emotions are often not that clear-cut, nor are they things that we either have or don't have. In addition, some people feel things more intensely or are better at handling and timing appropriate emotionally driven behaviour than others.

Many girls and women with ADHD say that they find it hard to understand, restrain, or tolerate their emotions, and often act in a way that leaves them feeling remorseful or ashamed. Much of living with ADHD is about getting to know yourself on the basis of your emotional register, trying to predict situations in which you normally encounter a rough patch, and finding new, more constructive ways of handling your emotions and their consequences.

Rejection-sensitivity dysphoria

It's probably safe to say that no one likes to get their mistakes and failures pointed out to them, and that social rejection and public criticism are associated with shame and embarrassment. But living with ADHD is often living a life where others continue to misunderstand and misinterpret your intentions. What by neurotypical people may be perceived as a gentle reminder or constructive feedback may then be perceived as a painful reminder or unjust criticism of an unfair reality. Furthermore, when difficulties regulating your emotional responses are at the core of your disability, it's even easier to imagine why so many females with ADHD describe unbearable pain and fear of perceived or actual rejection. Rejection-sensitive dysphoria (RSD) is commonly described as an intense and painful short-lived emotion, triggered by a real or perceived experience of rejection, criticism, or teasing. RSD may be as difficult for the person experiencing it to understand and handle as for the people around her to relate to. Many feel ashamed and embarrassed after a sudden emotional outburst or start to avoid social situations in which they might fail or be criticized altogether. Many also describe how their already low self-esteem is gradually deteriorating, leaving them in endless rumination about situations where they have felt attacked, criticized, or made a fool of, and how negative expectations adversely affect their relationships.

E AND THE EMOTIONAL COLDNESS

As a teenager, E realized she couldn't trust her instincts. Her feelings were so strong, her life and relationships always so intense and dramatic. While others were able to adapt their emotional volume, E always plunged into emotional turmoil.

She was often told that she should 'stop being such a drama queen' and stop stealing other people's space. Compounding this was the way her emotions could switch in a heartbeat, as if she could never be fully confident about how she would feel the next day, or even the next hour. She would find herself constantly cancelling things that she and her friends had planned.

Soon, her friends stopped counting on her turning up, or wanting to hang out with her. Advice that she should 'listen to her gut feeling' or 'just do what feels right in the moment' completely missed the mark. E felt that she had no gut feeling; or rather, that she had a thousand, often competing, gut feelings.

E gave up on the idea that emotions were her thing. Listening to her emotions was a luxury that she just couldn't indulge in. For years, E lived according to an ideal that she had created by studying people around her who seemed successful and happy. She constructed a system for when to eat, work out, and study. Activities involving social situations were risky and not that enjoyable, so were given no place in her routine life.

To her family and friends, it seemed as though E had finally grown out of her emotional turmoil and got her life in order. But E felt increasingly lonely and empty.

It wasn't until E sought help for her chronic depression and underwent an ADHD assessment that she started to properly connect with her emotions. After discovering that ADHD made it harder not only to regulate her attention but also to understand and control her emotions, E was gradually able to explore the rich life inside her.

Today, E takes care to notice and identify her emotions before deciding how to act on them. She has developed a system for 'flagging' feelings and emotional experiences and for calibrating their strength and intensity based on how they feel in the rest of her body. Doing this, she has successively developed her gut feeling that the rest of her friends, she says, seem to have got for free.

Thanks to her improved and more effective emotional regulation, E's self-esteem and self-confidence have also begun to blossom, so she now feels that she lives a full, rich life in sync with her ADHD.

R AND THE RESTLESS TEDIUM

Even if strong emotions often land girls and women with ADHD in trouble, the inability to tolerate boredom is what most consider their greatest problem.

'I've got a phobia about being bored,' R tells me, adding that she'd do almost anything to be spared the feeling of restlessness and emptiness that descends on her when there isn't something constantly catching her attention.

'I've caused so much unnecessary havoc and conflict simply because I can't stand being alone and bored. It's so unfair, because I really need to rest, but I just can't hack it.'

R makes sure that she's always occupied with something, tiring out her brain and body with exercise and work during the day so that she crashes in bed at night. This strategy worked well until recently, when repetitive stress injuries from all her physical activity started to set in. R is only in her early forties, and although she's so weary in both body and mind, she gets no peace and quiet in which to relax. She has found no other way than tiring herself out to the point of fatigue.

After a second period of sick leave for burnout, she was examined and diagnosed with ADHD. This has helped her to understand herself better and develop new tools to find rest and relaxation.

R, who had already tried countless relaxation techniques such as mindfulness and yoga, found an increased understanding of her inherited ADHD difficulties when she underwent a treatment programme for stress and emotional regulation. Afterwards, she was able to be more patient and respectful towards herself. Or as R with her droll self-irony put it: 'If anyone else had told me to sit staring at a raisin for quarter of an hour without also informing me that it's light-years more difficult for us with ADHD, I'd have shoved that f***ing raisin down their throat.'

Raisin meditation aside, her medication also made a huge difference. This, together with the fact that the treatment programme for burnout was ADHD-adapted, helped her to actually benefit from her treatment this time.

The shame and the life secret

Many girls and women with ADHD say that they have always felt different, sometimes alienated, from others from an early age. For many, this insight is a life secret that must on no account slip out. No one must know that they are flawed.

The protection of this secret becomes an ordeal from which

they get no rest. This heart-rending experience of trying to protect a secret vulnerability is often intimately associated with feelings of shame, which for many lead to fatigue, despair, and burnout.

Shame is one of our basic emotions that can stop us from saying and doing things that risk ostracism. There are subtle but distinct differences between guilt and shame. Guilt is a feeling we experience when we've done something wrong. It is painful but we can purge it by serving some form of punishment or repairing the damage we caused.

Shame, on the other hand, is associated with our intrinsic selves being flawed. This feeling of being aberrant or defective is thus intimately tied to our value as humans and our own existence. Shame can be based on a notion that we are unworthy or don't fit into a group, that we behave or think in an unorthodox way, or that we're simply wrong. Understanding shame in this way makes it easy to understand why the secret of being different, experienced by so many with ADHD, must be kept hidden at all costs.

Often, it's not the actual experience of shame we witness in others, but rather the strategies and behaviours they employ to get rid of painful feelings of shame.

Perhaps the relief that many girls and women feel when receiving their ADHD diagnosis is due to their being given a valid explanation for their problems directly related to some of the brain's most important functions. The insight of not being alone in this is often also a relief, allowing many to stand tall and feel a tenderness towards themselves and a sense of pride at having done all right after all, despite a lifelong uphill struggle.

There are many direct consequences of living with ADHD that can give rise to feelings of guilt and shame.

H AND THE HOUSEHOLD FINANCES

My husband and I have a very equal relationship, the same level of academic education, and roughly the same income. We share most of the costs but for practical reasons we decided that I would take care of the normal day-to-day household costs, while my husband spends pretty much the same amount every month on our mortgages and insurances.

The problem is that I've never been able to handle money. As soon as money goes into my account, I can feel it almost burning, and I get such strong impulses to buy stuff. And I don't mean stuff just for myself. I keep buying toys and gadgets for our kids and things for my husband and I just love spending and seeing their faces when I come home with some new surprise or other.

I also do a lot of online shopping when I get bored. This is rarely a wise thing to do, but for some reason I just can't stop myself. I've often ended up in situations where my money runs out before the end of the month. Usually, I've been able to borrow from my parents and siblings, but in the past few months I've taken a couple of SMS loans and they're really expensive. I was able to hide it from my husband until just recently but it came to light when I couldn't afford shoes and underwear for the children.

In one way, I feel so ashamed, but in another way, it's such a relief not to have to lie any more. In order never to end up in such a humiliating situation again, my husband and

I have agreed that the best thing would be for us to swap financial roles. With an automatic monthly transaction for our fixed costs debited from my account as soon as I get my paycheck, we're no longer jeopardizing the family's finances and our children's quality of life. We also realized that it is much easier for my husband to plan and organize the daily running of the household and the household costs.

We can spare the money that's left after the fixed costs have been deducted from my salary, and I don't have to feel ashamed when I get my impulses to do this illogical, rash purchasing to surprise my family. In fact, they often appreciate it too!

Chapter 6

Comorbidity – Life Is Not Fair

Living with ADHD will impose a lifelong vulnerability to both mental and physical comorbidity for many. In fact, a majority of children with ADHD, of both sexes, will struggle with other psychiatric diagnoses or conditions in addition to their ADHD.[1] For adults with ADHD, comorbidity will also be the rule rather than the exception, and about 80 per cent will have at least one other psychiatric diagnosis along with their ADHD.[2]

Much of the comorbidity – or other psychiatric conditions – associated with ADHD can be attributed to a combination of an underlying biological vulnerability (shared genetic factors) and how personal and situational circumstances are affected by the diagnosis. Even though feelings of shame may not be a direct cause of depression and anxiety, it's easy to imagine that they do not help if someone is already biologically predisposed to these conditions.

ADHD isn't a condition that we can simply detect and then cure. Comorbidity, however, can be. That's one of the reasons why a thorough ADHD assessment should always include a proper differential diagnostic perspective. Through a holistic view, we can tailor the proper accommodations, support, and treatment for every unique individual.

Comorbidity across life

The probability that girls and women with diagnosed or undiagnosed ADHD will need support from the healthcare and psychiatric services at some point during their life is high. Perhaps they have already knocked on the door of their local clinic at least once when they felt themselves losing their grip. Perhaps they needed someone to talk to, someone to help them understand why their brain simply refuses to obey and do what is best for them.

Having to ask others for help with problems can be fraught with shame. Admitting to yourself and others that you are in need of psychiatric care is not often something people boast about. It seems as if diagnoses and disorders that do not have a clear or simple aetiology – that can manifest differently in people and are associated with difficulties regulating emotions and behaviours – are usually subject to disparagement and stigmatization. ADHD is one such diagnosis.

Many girls and women with ADHD will testify to this and report feeling rejected, mistreated, and challenged by others, even healthcare services.

ADHD, anxiety, and mood disorders

Anxiety and depression are the most common psychiatric diagnoses in females in general, and girls and women with ADHD are at especially high risk of developing these disorders.

In fact, they live with an up to ten times higher risk of anxiety, mood disorders, and bipolar disorder during their lifespan compared to their non-ADHD peers, with the greatest risk during adolescence.[3]

It is common for females to have sought professional help countless times for general anxiety, depression, mood swings, and lethargy before they are referred for an ADHD assessment and get a diagnosis. Whether or not their anxiety and depression is attributable to undetected ADHD, these symptoms increase the likelihood of a diagnosis being overlooked.[4]

Of course, not all anxiety and depression, mood swings, and emotional outbursts in girls and women derive from misunderstood ADHD. However, primary anxiety disorders and mood disorders such as major depression or bipolar disorder often respond well to evidence-based treatment with cognitive behavioural therapy (CBT) and/or antidepressant or mood-stabilizing medication. But when the general anxiety and emotional dysregulation are better explained by the female manifestation of hyperactivity and impulsivity, there is a serious risk of these methods failing. And when it's not depression but the all-pervasive fatigue and amotivation that hits many girls with ADHD in puberty, antidepressants and CBT often have very little effect if the ADHD is not also addressed.

Unfortunately, many girls and women with ADHD are still undiagnosed or misdiagnosed, receiving little or incorrect treatment. Studies of US children with ADHD show that it is three times more common for girls with ADHD to have been prescribed antidepressant medication prior to their ADHD diagnosis compared to same-aged boys.[5] This saddening reality is likewise reflected in the finding that half as many girls as boys are actually treated for ADHD once properly diagnosed, causing unnecessary suffering and equally unnecessary costs for society.[6]

M AND THE GREAT DARKNESS

Today, M is a middle-aged woman. She has a family and many would probably describe her as a confident person with a successful career. But it hasn't always been like this. Nor is it how M tends to regard herself.

M tells me that she has always been an anxious type, a claim that stands out in sharp contrast against the image of the brave and outgoing woman others see. As a child, she was afraid of the dark and could lie awake at night worrying that her parents might get a divorce or that they or her siblings would leave her or die. Existential thoughts would spin round and round in her head, especially at night or when she wasn't occupied with other things.

As a girl, she learned that there was no point talking about these big questions that occupied her night. No one knew the answer to them anyway, and no one seemed to understand the sheer scale of her fears. At some point in her teens, things started to get really tough for M. Her ruminations about life and death and her fear of the dark had eased off a bit, only to be replaced by an all-consuming fatigue – what M calls 'the great darkness'.

'There were times when I just lay there, unable to haul myself out of bed. Even just raising my arm to brush my hair was too much for me. I had no starter motor, no spark plug. I had no energy to do anything.'

When M was a teenager, she would go once a week to see a pleasant, well-meaning older lady and discuss the causes of her fatigue. It was soon established that M was probably suffering from deep depression. She'd been such a kind, docile young girl. What could have happened to trigger this serious condition?

M and the therapist searched her childhood for explanations. What did that anxiety of hers represent? How was her relationship with her parents? M had never been particularly close to either her mother or father, but she had never regarded them as unusually bad parents either. However, over the years M and the therapist teased out a tangled, pained picture of her relationship with them. Had M perhaps never really felt that her parents had accepted her and appreciated her for who she was? Had they not been unusually preoccupied with their own careers? Why had no one comforted her about her existential ruminations? And when as a teenager and young adult she tried to find her own way in life, hadn't they been overly protective, hindering M from becoming an independent person?

After a couple of years of therapy, M broke off contact with her parents. They were aghast. Had they been completely blind and misguided? They thought they were helping M explore her independence despite her difficulties. Had they put their daydreaming daughter on the wrong track when trying to support her in her studies and her relationships? They were devastated, and remained estranged for years.

'Now I have become a mother of a little girl who's so much like me, it makes me wonder if it really was Mum and Dad who caused that crash in my teens. I also can't help but think that I was quite fortunate to get so much support from them during my chaotic teenage years. They were very involved in my life back then, which was difficult when my friends were so much more independent. But I often think that I've done all right anyway, in spite of the great darkness. Maybe this is at least in part due to my parents never entirely letting go of me.'

These days, M has the great darkness under control. She still calls it that, even though she knows, after receiving her ADHD diagnosis, that it was always about the trouble she had controlling her energy levels. At times when external structures offer no help, like when she's travelling with work or on holiday, she can still feel the great darkness lurking around the corner.

The difference today is that she knows that her fatigue is not something she can deal with by resting more. Rather, she needs to be her own inner, empathetic, no-nonsense mother, who takes little M by the hand and gently asks her to get up out of bed. The same inner voice that often will have to step up and gently whisper, 'Enough now, honey; put down your work, have something to eat, and go to bed. There is another day tomorrow as well.'

ADHD or borderline personality disorder?

As we have heard now, females with ADHD commonly describe intense feelings and rapid mood swings. However, as also discussed previously, emotional dysregulation is not included in the formal diagnostic criteria of ADHD but sometimes other diagnoses, such as borderline personality disorder, are considered in the differential diagnostic

discussion in an ADHD assessment. The overlap between
the two distinct disorders is common – both disorders can
appear in the same person, and research shows that they
share common genetic risk factors.[7] That really should come
as no surprise to us, since we know that largely the same or
closely associated brain networks are involved in regulating
emotions, mood, and attention.[8]

Thus, it is easy to imagine how tricky it can be to differentiate
between the two disorders. For most girls and women,
borderline issues develop at the onset of adolescence,
while ADHD has a childhood onset. Women with borderline
personality disorder also struggle with their own identity
and feel uncertain about both how they and others see
themselves. Intense, dramatic, and unstable relations, and an
extreme fear of abandonment are core features of borderline
personality disorder, since feelings about others change
quickly from extreme closeness to total rejection. Indeed,
many facets of life tend to change rapidly, impulsively, and
dramatically between extremes. To constantly view the world
as all good, or all bad, and to change interests and core
values rapidly is often as exhausting and frightening for those
affected as for people close to them. Many individuals with
borderline personality disorder describe all-consuming and
chronic feelings of inner emptiness, and some even struggle
with self-harm and recurring suicidal ideation.

While those with borderline personality disorder in many
ways will describe more extreme symptoms and greater
impairment of emotional dysregulation, it is obvious that the
two disorders have a distinct biological aetiology involving the
ability to regulate some of our most fundamental functions
and behaviours. Importantly, both ADHD and borderline
personality disorder have very little to do with morals, values,
talent, or willpower. As a young woman with both ADHD and

borderline personality disorder put it: 'If you'd been put in a car where the gas pedal and brakes are disconnected and out of sync, how easy do you think you'd find it to drive that car?'

Emotional instability with abrupt swings between hope and despair are alarming, confounding, and exhausting for others. Even if the most extreme mood swings aren't one of the ADHD diagnostic criteria, it's more the rule than the exception for girls and women to identify these very problems as being among the most disabling aspects of their condition.

Feelings of inner emptiness and alienation, and difficulties in defining a distinct identity are shared by ADHD and borderline personality disorder. Perhaps growing up with a feeling of being different without understanding why, and constantly having their feelings and emotions invalidated will do that to a person?

ADHD or autism?

In the neuropsychological assessment of ADHD, the team should also consider if someone displays symptoms that cannot be directly attributed to ADHD. If so, they need to determine the scope of those symptoms and whether they might better be understood within the parameters of another diagnosis. Often, they need to assess if any traits of autism need to be highlighted for the individual picture to be complete.

According to the former diagnostic manual DSM-IV, ADHD and autism could not be diagnosed in the same person. However, it has been clear both to patients and clinicians for a long time that this is not true. More realistically, about 30 per cent of girls and women with ADHD will also present with features of autism to different degrees.[9] Someone with autism typically has difficulties interpreting other people's social behaviour and expressing themselves in a way that allows others to understand what they mean, feel, and need. But different displays of hyperactivity and inattention – issues that lie at the heart of ADHD – may also cause everyday difficulties commonly attributed to autistic traits. Indeed, ADHD quite often causes problems when socializing with others. If, for example, you struggle with serious inattentiveness, it's no surprise that you miss important social signals, causing you to say or do inappropriate things. And if daydreaming and mind-wandering constantly steer your attention away from ongoing conversations or instructions given by others, you will probably often feel stupid, or perhaps get teased for not keeping up. This, of course, would be frustrating and awkward for anyone, but can be especially so for girls surrounded by people who tend to expect more developed social skills from them than from their male peers. Many girls and women with ADHD admit to the discomfort caused by feeling a social failure and being 'wrong' in social contexts, causing them to withdraw. They describe feeling 'totally exhausted' after social gatherings, even after being with people they like, and often need time for themselves to 'recharge'.

Difficulties with emotional regulation are common in ADHD and autism and can make social situations and interaction with others difficult. Strong, intense feelings take their toll, both on the person experiencing them and on the people receiving them.

Furthermore, liking and living by rituals and routines – often interpreted by others as possessing the rigid, inflexible behaviour common in autism – can also be the result of inattention and impulsivity. Perhaps you have realized that you can't trust your gut feeling and impulses and perhaps it becomes clear that planning, organizing, and prioritizing won't come naturally to you? The strategy then to overcompensate and create rigid rules and routines around most things in life may be a reasonable sacrifice.

Thus, the stress and avoidance of social situations could also be the consequences of ADHD rather than autism. However, if you already have one neurodevelopmental diagnosis, such as ADHD, you are more likely to also have other psychiatric diagnoses.

Social anxiety, OCD, or GAD?

Many teenagers and young adults seeking an ADHD assessment have previously been diagnosed with social anxiety or generalized anxiety disorder (GAD). For some, these diagnoses are the best explanatory models, while for others an underlying ADHD could be a better explanatory model and place to start.

As recently discussed, social situations demand a great deal from our executive attention. Many brain networks and processes need to harmonize, like a finely tuned orchestra under the baton of the frontal lobes, before we know how to behave in social contexts. In fact, the entire orchestra must play in concert for us to perform a seamless social symphony without making others puzzled or uncomfortable. As for so many other contexts where the ADHD brain fails us, it really doesn't matter how well each musician or instrument plays if we can't coordinate them to perform the piece that the audience expects from us.

If you, like many with ADHD, find it hard to remain attentive, coordinate your perceptions, calibrate your emotions, and curb your verbal impulsivity, small talk and mingling can pose a serious challenge. Distress at the possibility of messing up or a disproportionate fear of being judged or misunderstood can, of course, be a matter of generalized or social anxiety, or a precursor to it. But it could also be the outcome of a prudent strategy adopted by someone who knows she has serious difficulties staying attentive during a conversation or who has a history of making social faux pas. This is a reasonable strategy to avoid embarrassment.

If, on top of this, we can't really trust our autopilot to fully coordinate and perform what are automatic everyday behaviours to most, we may walk around with persistent anxiety, not unlike that described in GAD. Worry and anxiety over something that could go wrong almost always causes physiological reactions such as muscle tension, stiff neck, recurring headaches, or insomnia. To protect ourselves against this nagging feeling of anxiety, we may develop obsessive-compulsive traits and perfectionism, playing out a cycle that takes a great toll on our quality of life and mental health.[10] But if we recognize that we can be forgetful, perhaps we really did forget to unplug the iron, switch off the stove, or blow out those candles. In that case, everyday OCD-like rituals may be a smart survival strategy, at least until we have a more sophisticated explanatory model through an ADHD diagnosis.

ADHD, eating disorders, and body image

If we ask a female with ADHD about their dietary habits and how they feel about their bodies, roughly 10 per cent will admit to having struggled with an eating disorder at some point in their life.[11] An even larger proportion, probably a little over half of them, will also say that they're still constantly unhappy with their bodies and use food as a means of regulating energy levels and emotions.

Furthermore, ADHD is over-represented among overweight girls, and the physical problems that accompany obesity are common among children and adults with ADHD.[12] Knowing what we know about ADHD, this is not particularly surprising. ADHD is related to problems regulating brain levels of dopamine, which is also involved in the regulation of hunger and satiety.

Living with ADHD means a susceptibility to dopamine triggers, such as alcohol, drugs, sex, gambling, and shopping. An association between ADHD and both eating disorders and obesity is also apparent.

Unfortunately, insomnia is also the rule rather than the exception in ADHD, and interrupted sleep can give rise to weight gain. When we are stressed and unable to get a proper night's sleep, our bodies release stress- and appetite-stimulating hormones such as cortisol and leptin, to store energy. This is a clever survival mechanism to increase the body's fat reserves, improving our chances of survival in times of uncertainty or danger. However, as living with ADHD by many is described as living a life where stress and insomnia are the rule rather than the exception, difficulties regulating hunger, satiety, and weight maintenance may be ever present.

The impulsivity of ADHD makes it hard for many to resist the temptations of sweets and calorie-dense food. Also, the inattentiveness and the difficulties identifying and regulating feelings of hunger and satiety will cause problems in trying to maintain a regular, healthy diet. Perhaps you are one of many with ADHD who gets so caught up in things that you forget to eat, only to find yourself starving and lethargic hours later. At this point, your body will crave carbohydrates, fat, salt, and sweets, quickly and in abundance. In this state, it's almost impossible to plan and prepare a well-balanced menu. Instead, you grab a bag of sweets, a sandwich, chips, fast food, or a sweet fizzy drink. The hours of fasting are replaced by a feeding frenzy of carbohydrates and calories, usually way over your recommended daily intake.

Or perhaps you are one of many with ADHD caught up in endless cycles of yo-yo dieting, alternating self-starvation and binging, where temporary weight loss is followed by sustained weight gain? One might think that children grow out of this kind of behaviour in their teens, but many women with ADHD describe the shame in still not having control over their eating habits.

We all comfort-eat now and then. A relationship has ended, someone's been dumped, so down goes the spoon into a tub of ice-cream. A friend fails you, so you turn to Netflix, chips, and chocolate.

For many women, their ADHD imposes problems in understanding, tolerating, and containing their emotions. These difficulties in articulating and offloading emotions may also be a reason to self-medicate with food. When it comes down to it, food is legal and eating is often seen as a much less drastic act than drinking alcohol or taking drugs. The problems overeating can cause, however, can be just as serious.

One might think that grief, shame, or anger would be the most common emotional triggers of binge eating. Interestingly, however, being bored is by all accounts by far the most common cause of overeating in both children and adults with ADHD. Not infrequently, a sense of being under-stimulated and not knowing what to do will lead to a restless rummaging through the fridge.

Perhaps you are one of many with ADHD who is a quick eater, shovelling food without even savouring the taste, noticing only when it's too late that you're stuffed? One fascinating theory is that the difference in perception and body signals commonly described in ADHD results in different sensations of hunger and satiety. Further, according to this theory, the ADHD brain may register the amount of energy ingested with a delay. In other words, the signals of how much food you have consumed reach your ADHD brain slower than in those without the diagnosis.[13]

One recurring point I will make in this book concerning all the possible theories and the different adverse behaviours and outcomes in ADHD is also highly relevant for the association between weight gain, eating disorders, and ADHD – namely that ADHD has very little to do with someone's morals, character, or poor judgement. Rather, living with ADHD makes it harder to regulate emotions and behaviours in spite of knowing what is right and good for you. Hunger and satiety are no exception. To start tackling these problems you need an understanding of how your ADHD brain works, rather than a few well-meaning lectures on nutrition.

H AND THE GREAT HUNGER

H was once a happy, carefree, little girl. She had a big appetite and her parents often had to restrict her meals and hide away tempting treats. But it was not until her teens – after some snide comment from a boy in her class – that H herself began to think of her eating as a problem. She decided to go on a diet. However, that strategy did not turn out successfully.

First, she tried skipping breakfast, but that just made it even harder for her to concentrate at school. Whereas before she could at least stay focused until lunch, even her morning lessons now became a perfect parade of mind-wandering and daydreaming. Moreover, she was so hungry by lunchtime that she would wolf her food down in the school canteen, giving boys even more opportunity to comment on her voracious appetite.

So, H started to skip school lunches too; they were associated with too much shame and embarrassment. Not to mention PE classes. Aware of her burgeoning weight, every minute in the gym bordered on torture for H, who had always loved moving around, swimming, and playing outdoors.

Since she felt observed and judged when eating, H concluded that the only way to eat undisturbed was to sneak home after school and gobble down as much as she could before her parents came home. At least now she herself was the only witness to her humiliation and shame.

At the age of 14, H saw a clip about eating disorders on YouTube. She figured that since everything else she tried had failed, purging may be the solution. She began throwing up the food she had binged in secret. At first, she lost weight, but pretty soon her weight plateaued and started to go up again. Then she realized she really had a problem. The daily vomiting left her weak and exhausted, and keeping it from her parents and friends was extremely time consuming.

After a while, her parents realized that something was off with H. She couldn't keep herself together any more and started staying home from school; some days she could barely get out of bed. Her entire world circulated around eating, cravings, and her repulsion towards her own body. At this point, H had admitted her problems to her parents and she wanted help. Her parents contacted a clinic for eating disorders. She visited the clinic off and on for a few years, but nothing really changed. She did have periods where she managed to resist her impulses to eat, but it soon tipped over into anorexia.

'Half my childhood and my entire adolescence was defined by my eating disorders,' says H laconically. And no treatment helped – until her therapist at the clinic suggested an ADHD assessment. Her ADHD diagnosis turned out to be the missing piece of the puzzle and marked the beginning of a deeper understanding of herself.

H admits that her relationship to food still isn't totally uncomplicated, but she no longer has an eating disorder. She can eat what she wants, as long as she stays within certain limits. Her first and most important rule is to eat regularly at all times. She makes sure always to eat three meals a day and three snacks, with a hearty breakfast in the morning. And she avoids fast carbohydrates on an empty stomach but allows herself sweets and desserts after a well-balanced meal. She also goes easy on the alcohol, since she noticed that it increases her appetite and weakens impulse control. When she sticks to these routines, she can treat herself to things on which she once binged, and she no longer feels that her life is dictated by food.

Alcohol, drugs, and addiction

Having ADHD is associated with a risk of numerous adverse consequences, and for some adolescents with ADHD, a tendency to experiment with tobacco, alcohol, and drugs will develop into harmful use and addiction.[14]

Indeed, research shows that ADHD is a risk factor for developing an addiction to alcohol and illicit drugs, but why is that and what exactly does it mean? Is it the consequence of negative attention from adults, misguided interventions in school, failed friendships, or the result of reoccurring childhood trauma? Or is it a kind of self-medication for ADHD symptoms of restlessness and impulsivity that increases the risk of addiction to alcohol or drugs?

Thanks to an increasing body of scientific literature, we can say with certainty that the correlation between ADHD and hazardous substance use and addiction is largely attributable to a shared genetic predisposition. As previously discussed, ADHD is highly affected by inherited factors. This is true also for substance use disorders. Consequently, we could expect a strong association between ADHD and addiction.[15]

Importantly, however, this does not mean that everyone with ADHD will become an alcoholic or drug addict, but rather that they probably have an increased susceptibility. Those living with ADHD need to be extra careful around substances that for everyone could result in addiction or substance use disorders.

W AND THE WINE

W looks back at her teenage self and shudders. She says she often gets cold, icy feelings when she thinks about the incredible risks she exposed herself to when she started drinking alcohol at the age of 13. Fairly soon after her first experience with alcohol, she and her friends devoted a lot of time to planning weekend parties. It was a thrill to find ways to steal wine and spirits from the parents' drinks cabinets or entice older siblings to purchase it for them, and to think up clever ways to avoid being caught. But it wasn't long before it was obvious that something set W apart from her friends.

'It was like I never had an inner thermostat for when to stop drinking. The others quickly learned from their mistakes, but I just kept on getting totally wasted. At first, my friends mostly just laughed at me, but soon they started to think I was a burden and an embarrassment when they have to look after me. And I'd do so many stupid things that I'd never would have done sober. I'd cringe with shame afterwards, but still end up doing the same thing the next weekend. And the next, and the next. And it wasn't just embarrassing things, either. Incredibly reckless and dangerous things happened, too, when I was under the influence of alcohol. I had unprotected sex with guys I didn't know. I'd sometimes get so hammered that I'd have no idea where I woke up or what had happened before I'd crashed out. I rode around drunk on a moped and once we nicked a car and drove it into a lake.'

As an adult, such foolhardy adolescent transgressions seem remote to W, but she still hasn't developed that thermostat that tells her how much she can drink without losing control. She realizes that she probably was born with a greater sensitivity to the effects of alcohol and therefore takes better care of herself nowadays. 'I use alcohol more moderately now and I think that I keep a closer eye on myself and my reactions than others who don't have ADHD do. And I never drink when I'm off balance, on an empty stomach, or in situations where I need to be in full control, such as work settings.'

W has also made sure to talk to her own children about the propensity for hazardous alcohol use that the family has inherited. As an adult, she discovered that both her maternal grandparents had had alcohol problems, and that this was the reason why her own mother never touched alcohol.

C AND THE CANNABIS

After years of nagging and pressure from parents, friends, and boyfriends, C sought help at an addiction clinic for young adults. She was 14 when she tried marijuana for the first time and she remembers it as if it were yesterday (quite the achievement since her memories of the following ten years are neither clear nor uplifting). But for C it was the first time that something actually worked for her lifelong insomnia and that ever-present buzzing of thoughts in her head.

She lost count of how many times she and her parents went to the child and adolescent psychiatric clinic, of how many ineffective drugs and explanations she was given before she finally found her solution with cannabis.

'It was wonderful. It went all quiet in my head and all my agitation just dissolved. When I smoked, I could go to sleep at a normal time, and at first, I even started to do better at school. I shed that restlessness that made lessons so horrible, and my self-confidence improved. When Mum and Dad dragged me off to the social services it was as if they wanted to deprive me of the only thing that kept me going, without replacing it with anything else. After all, I'd tried all their treatments already. I already knew it wasn't going to work for me.'

C smoked cannabis almost daily for ten years. At the beginning, she didn't notice much of a difference between herself and her non-smoking friends. Later on, she didn't care. She made a few failed attempts to quit on her own and to get help but soon lost motivation and went back to the old way of dealing with stuff.

'Everyone wanted to help, but no one understood the underlying problem. But in the end, it became obvious, even to me, that there was no way forward except quitting. My friends had moved on in life, left home, started studying, or got a job. I ploughed on with temping jobs and sinking self-esteem. The smoking wasn't helping that much either any more and I was constantly angst-ridden and low. Yet, I couldn't stop, because then I had to face up to everything I'd messed up and everyone I'd let down.'

Besides nicotine and alcohol, cannabis is the most common drug on which people with ADHD get addicted. Many find, just like C, that it's effective for the symptoms of ADHD at first. For C, learning about her ADHD was an important part of the puzzle en route to kicking the habit. Once she had pulled herself together and sought help for what she suspected was ADHD, she had the fortune to find herself at a clinic that didn't reject her for her cannabis addiction; on the contrary, they understood that the underlying

ADHD was a risk factor for ending up where C had. They used C's own motivation to undergo an ADHD assessment as a driving force to become drug-free and initiated the assessment while she was recovering from her dependency. Just this – the simple fact of something actually in motion – was in itself a powerful and important motivational factor in defeating the substance use disorder.

Maybe it's not all ADHD's fault?

For some women with ADHD, the greatest problem or suffering isn't primarily due to their ADHD. Previous life experiences and distinct comorbidities can, for many, bear an even greater responsibility for their disabilities in everyday life, and only a fraction of their more complex situation can be attributed to their ADHD.

For some women, personality disorders, addiction, destructive relationships, or untreated depression will explain far more of their current impairments than ADHD. Again, it is central that assessment and interventions aim to focus on a possible ADHD diagnosis, as well as identify and describe how individual psychosocial factors or comorbidities contribute to the unique situation. Simply saying that someone does or doesn't have ADHD doesn't help them deal with other problems if they're not described and factored into treatment and accommodations.

Thus, all girls and women must be treated – pharmacologically and therapeutically – based on their entire symptomology. ADHD treatment only will seldom solve other co-existing problems, such as a substance use disorder or a personality disorder. These distinct conditions should be dealt with alongside, or sometimes prior to, ADHD treatment.

Notes

1 Gillberg *et al.*, 2004
2 Nigg, 2013
3 Biederman *et al.*, 2012; Marangoni et al., 2015
4 Nadeau, 2002; Quinn & Madhoo, 2014
5 Quinn & Wigal, 2004
6 Castle *et al.*, 2007
7 Kuja-Halkola *et al.*, 2018; Matthies & Philipsen, 2014
8 Petrovic, 2015; Sanchez *et al.*, 2019
9 Kopp *et al.*, 2010; Gillberg, 2010
10 Arnold *et al.*, 2005
11 Nazar *et al.*, 2016
12 Cortese *et al.*, 2016; Cortese & Tessari, 2017
13 Kaisari *et al.*, 2018; Kurz *et al.*, 2017
14 Elkins *et al.*, 2018
15 Skoglund *et al.*, 2015; Skoglund *et al.*, 2014

Chapter 7

Living a Life with ADHD

N AND THE RESTARTS

'I'm so fed up with myself. I struggle 24 hours a day
to get things into some sort of blasted control. I live
with a constant feeling that it can't go on like this, that
something has to change, that something's missing, wrong,
needs fixing.

'I've lost count of all the times I've "started a new life".
All these constant restarts, where I go all in, proudly
proclaiming to everyone and anyone that I've found the
key, I've got the answer, I have the solution. Only to be back
at square one a couple of days later. And to sit there with
the shame burning my cheeks, with "told you so" looks in
other people's eyes and a sickening sense of dejection in
the pit of my stomach.

'Everyone who's tried to understand and help me says the
same thing: "You have such good self-insight, you already
know what you have to do, you've made such progress."
But they're wrong. I'm just so blasted verbal. I can
articulate things, experiences, and insights in a way that
makes others think I'm close to my goal. But nothing ever
changes. I tread on the same mines every single day. The

knowledge that I haven't found the way ahead this time either is so oppressive and humiliating. It's as if I can't trust myself or my instincts. It's frightening and depressing. I'm so fed up with myself.'

Poor executive functions due to ineffective communication between the frontal lobes and other brain areas cause problems for people with ADHD, both structurally and emotionally. Perhaps you are one of many women with ADHD who, due to this often-invisible disability, have to struggle so much harder than others just to get by? Has your ADHD interfered with almost everything in your life, including your ability to establish and maintain even the most basic routines and habits? You are not alone, and it is not uncommon for girls and women to describe their lives as a series of perpetual restarts with a growing sense of being on the wrong track without having a strategy to turn to. Many also suspect – probably rightly so – that society has higher expectations on them than on their male brothers, partners, or colleagues.

T AND TYPICAL FEMALENESS

T sailed through school. In hindsight, she believes it was because she so often managed to zigzag her way forward by predicting what friends, teachers, and parents expected from her. Thanks to strong social and verbal skills, she usually did what was expected of her. And she got good marks until her last year of secondary school, when the demands grew heavier as she was required to function more independently. As she began to lag behind, she also was struck by what she called 'the massive fatigue'.

After countless visits to her family doctor, blood tests, and examinations, it was concluded that T was probably depressed. She was told that she shouldn't put such high demands on herself, that she should relax more and have some fun rather than just bury herself in her studies. T says that her depression diagnosis never really made sense to her. She was never depressed back then. Now, 25 years later, she certainly can be. As an adult, she has been what she describes as clinically depressed for long periods at a time. But back when she was a teenager, her symptoms didn't have a depressive quality. She felt more as if she was absolutely drained of energy.

In hindsight, she could see that her ADHD symptoms were there all along. She had never been able to concentrate properly for that long or read a book from beginning to end. But she always came up with clever ways to get around it. In class, she'd stay alert and awake by sitting at the front, constantly asking questions, or being in dialogue with teachers and classmates, creating vivid, artistic note-taking systems and fidgeting with her hands, feet, and hair. To cover up for difficulties with concentration and reading, she downloaded audio books, and watched films and YouTube clips, ensuring that she didn't miss any information that others gained from course literature and textbooks.

During secondary school, things got tougher, but T managed to keep her grades up by putting in all the effort she could. However, this made her so tired at the end of the day that she didn't have any energy left to drag herself to football. Hanging out with friends was not an option either. She'd spend the afternoons, evenings, and weekends trying to recharge her energy so that she could get up in the morning, when the struggle would start all over again. Only T really understood how hard she fought, how difficult it was to propel herself forward without a starting motor, spark plug, fuel, or throttle control.

T consulted a psychiatrist for the first time while on maternity leave, six months after having her first child, and feeling burnt out. The shame ate away at her when she tried to explain how she could feel so terrible just when life should be at its best. She had a lovely little family, a house with a garden, and the luxury of being able to take a whole year of leave with her daughter. But under the surface, her life was 'one hell of a mess'.

She hadn't yet built up any routines around her daughter's daytime feeding and sleeping requirements. The sleep deprivation and the stress around not being able to predict her daughter's constantly changing needs pushed her towards insanity. Her family and friends stepped in with well-meant but totally misdirected advice like: 'Don't make such high demands on yourself', 'Relax and enjoy these first months with your baby; you'll never get them back', 'Don't be such a control freak; no one expects you to be perfect.'

T just sat there crying. Not being more grateful for her life filled her with shame and fear. She felt that it would be better if she didn't exist. Gradually with her psychiatrist, she disentangled her situation. A cooperative puzzle emerged where T placed the pieces on the table and, together with the psychiatrist, tried to make them fit. A complex picture of coping strategies for symptoms of inattention and lacking executive functions slowly started to appear.

T had always known that she couldn't afford the luxury of trusting everyday things to fall into place or sort themselves out, and so had spent her entire life creating routines and rituals. Her family and friends were blind to how hard she'd struggled. In the early days of her relationship with baby L's father, she would often get small, loving comments about her idiosyncrasies and routines; nowadays, these peculiarities were mostly a source of antagonism and irritation.

T felt people thought that she was inflexible and egocentric, that she always had to get her own way. She was her harshest judge and she agreed with them. She often had veritable meltdowns if things didn't go as planned, if someone messed up her tidy house, if L got sick, or newly established routines were broken.

T's ADHD diagnosis was a watershed moment for her. Her behaviour became comprehensible to her, and she could gradually dismantle her defensive walls and find new, more rational strategies. But others still didn't see or understand the battle she had been fighting. She gave up trying to convince her parents, L's father, and her friends that she has a brain that's not wired the same way as theirs.

Their lack of understanding left her unhappy and dejected. And sometimes she partially agreed with them, wondering if she maybe faked her way to a diagnosis. Perhaps she was just lazy and found excuses for her failures and inabilities? Everyone thought parenthood was hard, right?

ADHD is a serious diagnosis with a good prognosis. It can result in substantial impairment and extensive comorbidity. Yet it is often invisible to others. However, when you understand how ADHD creates difficulties with prioritization, organization, and planning daily activities, as well as getting started with and finalising important tasks, assessing time, and remembering crucial appointments, it becomes easier to appreciate how ADHD makes motherhood stressful.

Indeed, women often tell us that their strategies for handling their impairments fail them when they become mothers. They were effective when they only had themselves to think about, but when the first-degree equation gets compounded into a second- or third-degree equation, not even the most sophisticated strategies may suffice. To make matters worse, many women feel that it isn't particularly healthy for a child or a family to have to adapt to the routines and strategies they have established for themselves over the years. But without them they often feel rudderless in a tempest that risks drowning the ones they love the most.

T described another side of ADHD that often poses a particular challenge to women in social situations. Many women feel a profound sense of shame at not being able to function as a woman, a partner, and a mother.

Any intimacy with baby L's father was out of the question, T said. They argued constantly and she simply couldn't stand being physically close to him on top of L's constant need for attention and closeness. T cleaned and cleaned their home, but her work was never done. It had evolved into a painful, vicious cycle, where she started cleaning one room, got stuck on another mess, and in the end the whole house was upside down without even the slightest hint of order.

T just wanted to order a skip, chuck everything in it, and start all over again. This, too, led to conflict with baby L's father, who called her insensitive and selfish for wanting to throw out his things as well.

On some days, she would get hooked up on some detail or other to the extent that she forgot to eat and check on her baby in her pram. A neighbour came over one day and told her crossly that little L had been lying screaming for over an hour in the pram. T looked down at her 1990s CD collection, ashamed under the reproachful eyes of her neighbour. 'What kind of mother am I?' she thought. When L's father came home from work, she was still there, bent over her CDs, frantically trying to order them by date of release, or no, by artist would be better, or no, by colour of the covers. She had seen people do this with their books, which sparked her to switch to the bookshelves.

Sensory processing and perception

Are you one of many women with ADHD who suspects that you experience physical sensations in a different way from others? Perhaps you have heard since you were young that, 'No, this doesn't hurt; you are just exaggerating' or, 'Don't you know when to stop; it's not normal to push yourself that hard'? Many with ADHD also say that they experience sensitivity around temperature, physical contact, gastrointestinal functions, how clothes feel against the body, and hunger or satiety.

However, little research has been done on why this is and not much is known that could explain and corroborate these prevalent testimonies. The same kind of aberrant bodily experiences are also common in people with autism.

For women with ADHD, these difficulties can be particularly problematic, not so much because they differ between men and women, but because of society's expectations – and sometimes those of women themselves – of female behaviour. Being sensitive to physical contact, touch, and clothing can be a challenge for a growing, changing body during puberty, pregnancy, and breastfeeding. Feeling discomfort when nursing often has nothing to do with the love or strength of the bond between mother and child. However, it's easy to misinterpret it in this way, and for the mother to feel guilt and shame at finding intimate contact with her baby stressful and intrusive. These feelings are often reinforced by ignorant or judgemental comments of others.

It's also common for people with ADHD to often bump into furniture, hurt themselves, spill and drop things. They feel clumsy and awkward. In fact, different kinds of motor impairments are common in ADHD, and, like so much else when it comes to our complicated brain, it's not exactly clear what causes these difficulties with coordination and fine or gross motor control. It is believed to be associated with brain networks including the cerebellum and the basal ganglia (see Chapter 2 on the brain).

Yet again, might we have reason to ask ourselves if we expect different things of girls and boys when it comes to these particular domains? Could fine motor difficulties be particularly challenging for girls, since they affect everything from handwriting, the ability to draw and perform hand crafts to table manners? Putting on makeup, doing hair, adjusting clothes, walking in heels, or dancing might not be things that all females want to do or value that highly, but for many girls and women with ADHD it's not even an option.

Support from a physiotherapist or occupational therapist can help and improve this situation for many. Also, for some, central stimulant medication may improve both coordination and precision difficulties due to ADHD-induced motor problems.

Sleeping difficulties – to have to get up just after dropping off

Even though they are not included in the diagnostic criteria, sleeping difficulties are very common in ADHD. Indeed, some kind of disordered sleep occurs in eight out of ten adults with ADHD.[1] Perhaps you are one of many women with ADHD unable to wind down in the evening due to whirling thoughts and sleep-disrupting anxiety? Or perhaps you are incapable of finding enough peace of mind to fall asleep because of hypersensitivity to sound or light, or how the sheets feel against the skin?

Poor quality of sleep or difficulties getting to sleep can cause health issues if prolonged. Daytime tiredness subverts work capacity and increases the risk of work-related accidents. A lack of sleep can also be a precursor to lifestyle-related ill-health and disorders, such as obesity and high blood pressure. Furthermore, insomnia or disrupted sleep increases your sensitivity to stress and susceptibility to mental health problems.[2] Many with ADHD will tell us that sleep has constantly eluded them, causing them unbearable problems that they deal with in destructive ways. Some will turn to alcohol, addictive medication, or drugs such as cannabis. What can seem like a clever solution at first will, however, almost always end up in a worse scenario. The likelihood of them needing more and more of the substance that provided initial relief is high, and an addiction can quickly develop.

Many adults with ADHD often hear themselves described as 'such a night owl' or 'a real pain to put to bed, ever since infancy'. Others hear from current partners that 'you move around like a propeller in your sleep' or 'it's almost impossible to wake you up in the mornings'. Furthermore, restless legs and feelings of inner restlessness when going to sleep are more common in ADHD compared with others without the diagnosis. And the link between ADHD and sleep is a two-way one – living with ADHD means there is an inherited risk of sleeping problems, and sleeping problems will inevitably exacerbate ADHD symptoms. Moreover, certain medications for ADHD can have sleeping problems as side-effects by virtue of their central-stimulating effects.

In summary, ADHD-related insomnia can have many causes, from restless legs to an innately different circadian rhythm, and is often one of the main problems, regardless of the underlying cause. Given the major impact sleeping problems have on quality of life, it is important to carefully evaluate individual sleep patterns in both ADHD assessment and treatment. In fact, different kinds of support and intervention for insomnia should often be a part of a complete ADHD treatment regimen.

J AND THE BRAIN THAT NEVER WANTED TO SLEEP

J's mother always said that she was a real challenge as a baby. To be sure, she was a little ray of sunshine, happy, alert, and curious. But she was also perpetually active and would never be calm or still. 'It was almost as if you were bored being an infant,' her mother often said and explained that she never wanted to sleep in her pram or cot. Once she had learnt to crawl and ultimately walk, she wasn't bored any more but now there were so many new things to discover and so little time to sleep. 'You didn't want to miss anything and the slightest noise or movement outside your pram would wake you up,' J's mother said. Soon enough, J's mother developed a hatred of external disturbances that could deprive J of sleep.

As a schoolgirl, J could be out until midnight. She rarely amassed the hours of sleep recommended for a girl of her age. J's mother and father never had any quality adult time together in the evenings when J was a baby, but it was the mornings during her school years that put the greatest strain on the family. J would sleep as if she were unconscious, and it often took over an hour to get her out of bed. With her parents desperate to get off to work, their mornings turned into pitched battles.

When she reached her teens, J's sleeping patterns became more in sync with those of her peers, but still at the age of 24, she was finding it just as hard to settle down at night and get up in the morning.

'My brain refuses to switch off. I just get loads of thoughts and ideas spinning around in my head and there's no way I can wind down and just let go. I've tried everything. I smoked marijuana and cigarettes every evening for a while, not for kicks or because I wanted to, but to shut up that damn buzzing head of mine. But eventually I got caught and had to go and leave urine samples every week and then it just wasn't worth using that shit any more. But it's still the only thing that has come even close to helping me – well, a little at least.

'I can't go on like this any more – I'll get the sack if I don't sort out my sleep. But once I've finally dropped off, I just can't get up. I never used to be depressed or down, but now I almost always feel low. I walk round as if in a fog throughout the days, just longing to go to bed. Excuse my language, but it's a f***ing nightmare, this. The irony of thinking about sleep all day long and then not being able to fall asleep when you finally crash into bed in the evening.'

After an ADHD assessment and diagnosis, J was prescribed the natural sleep hormone melatonin to establish a more normal sleep-wake cycle. It made her feel more naturally tired and made it easier to establish regular sleeping routines. The idea is that when daylight percolates through in the morning, the melatonin is broken down and we wake up refreshed after a good night's sleep and without the hangover effects of more potent and sometimes addictive drugs. J also tried out a 13-kilo weighted chain blanket, which improved her quality of sleep and reduced the number of times she woke up at night.

Procrastination – why do today what I can put off till tomorrow?

One of the main impairments in ADHD concerns the difficulties in self-control and sustained motivation. It may sound insignificant, and a common misconception is that it's merely a matter of will and character. Few things are further from the truth. Many women with ADHD will admit they know what has to be done but somehow find themselves totally unable to do the task, whether it be heaps of laundry, dirty dishes, work demands, or unpaid bills. This is hard, especially when it is looked on by others (and often also the person themselves) as general sloppiness, laziness, depression, or incompetence.

The question is whether we, as a society, find it even harder to put up with these kinds of problems in women than we do in men? We hear the term 'bachelor pad' and perhaps picture a room that is charmingly untidy, or at least less pedantically neat than what we may visualize when we think about a young woman's first flat. And isn't it still a little more remarkable when a grown-up woman turns up at work with her hair mussed and her blouse lopsidedly buttoned than when a man of a similar age swans into the meeting quarter of an hour late with bits of breakfast caught in his beard? Is it still the case, perhaps, that we expect more from women and mothers when it comes to keeping their lives together or doing loads of things simultaneously?

Watching clips on social media or reading articles in the media, we may see women pursuing a career focusing on their personal development and at the same time being an ever-present parent and a partner, having an attractive, well-toned body, and, of course, maintaining a nice, tidy home. But many women with ADHD find themselves unable to keep everyday things from getting out of hand, let alone remember to buy new seasonal clothes for the kids, bake for the school sale, or arrange social events for work. They find themselves falling short of society's description of a successful and responsible woman. Does this mean we expect women to manage all these different roles simultaneously more naturally than men?

D AND THE GROWING PILES OF WASHING UP

D was a particularly talented and wise woman who had lived her whole life without her ADHD diagnosis. She had tried countless antidepressants for her anxiety and rejected them all, and she had been given almost as many explanatory models for her social difficulties and professional debacles.

D felt lonely, flawed, and isolated. The thing making D's struggle so hard to understand for herself and others was that she was actually really socially gifted and one of the sharpest minds on her work team. And when she underwent her ADHD assessment as an adult, alternative explanations for D's loneliness and professional failures emerged.

D told me that during a previous therapy session for social anxiety she was advised to invite a colleague home after work. D explained to her therapist that her home was such a mess that such a home assignment was impossible. It would simply be too embarrassing to let anyone see the chaos that was her home back then. She was told by the well-intended therapist, 'No one really cares about those superficial things', and, 'It's the social interaction people focus on. A little messiness may only be disarming, helping others to relax.'

However, if the therapist had tried to find out more, it would have become clear that D probably did the right thing in not inviting anyone home given the state of it back then. The sink was full of dirty washing up that had accumulated over months. And since there were no clean plates to eat off, D had takeaway food every evening, the boxes for which she had carefully sorted but not taken to the recycling bins. They formed two gigantic walls by the living room door. Then there were all the boxes containing old stuff from a distant uncle that D hadn't got round to sorting out, as well as the broken TV and the two old fish tanks that hadn't seen any residents since the last salamander met its maker eight years ago.

D felt, and rightly so, that a visitor could easily get the wrong impression of her. And since she procrastinated around getting her home in an acceptable condition, her social life gradually dwindled – if invitations to social events can't be reciprocated, they tend to dry up.

A more productive psychological approach would have

factored in the problems D had controlling and influencing her motivational processes. It's also interesting to note that as her ADHD investigation came to an end and she received the right diagnoses, explanatory model, and treatment regimen with central stimulants and concrete occupational-therapeutic support, the piles of washing up and junk began to reduce in almost perfect correlation to increasing social activity.

Routines that build fences

Try to imagine having to live a life without shades of grey, where each 'not too much', 'maybe', 'I don't feel like it right now', and 'I'll do it tomorrow instead' risks bursting the banks to an uncontrolled chaos. One of the problems of living with ADHD is sometimes described as not being able to work with nuances or smaller, finer brushstrokes in life.

Do you, like many girls and women with ADHD, find it unduly difficult to prioritize what needs to be done now and what can wait until later? Or do you feel as if tasks, requests, and instructions get no natural distribution and just line up at the front of your mind, all demanding the same attention and memory capacity? For many, this can ramp up stress levels that others find hard to understand and handle. 'Come on, leave it. It can wait till tomorrow' or, 'Why waste so much energy on this? Forget it for now' and, 'Don't get worked up over that; it's not going to happen until next week.'

Many women with ADHD find the stress and uncertainty so difficult to stand that they make 'all or nothing' decisions. To make their lives work and hold everything together, they decide to *always* do *everything* in a certain way. No half-ways, no exceptions, no sleep-ins. Setting these extreme, non-negotiable bars around yourself can quickly turn your life into a prison. Once again others stand beside you looking puzzled. 'Take a break, for God's sake', 'You're completely exhausted', 'You need to be kinder to yourself.'

But as so many girls and women with ADHD testify, no exemption goes by unpunished. Beyond the prison walls lurks imaginary or assured chaos of insurmountable proportions. Best to stay behind the fence. At least control can be maintained there. And control is hard currency when you are living with ADHD.

Doubt – a constant companion

Many accounts of ADHD describe failing at life itself. Not fitting in. Living with a secret that has to be protected at all costs – the secret of being different. Many women will testify to the sadness and disappointment of having plucked up the courage to confide these feelings in a friend, parent, or partner only to be met with comments like, 'But we all feel like that now and again' or, 'I know; this stuff is hard for me, too.'

Since ADHD – like all the other psychiatric diagnoses in the *Diagnostic and Statistical Manual* DSM-5 – is a diagnosis based primarily on interviews and personal testimonies without verification through blood tests or X-rays, many regard ADHD as a less valid or reliable diagnosis. This can lead to people doubting their diagnosis, wondering if they over- or under-exaggerated their symptoms which led to an incorrect conclusion by the health professionals. It also makes many adults with ADHD sensitive about outside opinions regarding their diagnosis, and about their treatment.

Even though it's understandable that well-meaning families and friends want to normalize and include someone who feels different, it often backfires. In many cases, such as in adolescence, it can be helpful to normalize a teen's behaviour, waiting to see if difficulties or experiences develop. However, often this fundamentally sound strategy can also leave serious problems unidentified and untreated. It is a well-established truth that the earlier you receive a diagnosis for any disorder, the better chance you have of getting the right support to help avoid negative consequences. This seems to be true for physical as well as for psychiatric diagnoses, and ADHD is no exception.

Notes

1   Wynchank *et al.*, 2017; Wynchank *et al.*, 2018
2   Instanes *et al.*, 2018

Chapter 8

Family Life and Relationships

Nature or nurture?

In the last 20–30 years, we have learned from research that the risk of developing ADHD is heavily influenced by inherited factors and not, as previously believed, caused by poor or lax parenting, bad diets, or too much screen time. Indeed, approximately 80 per cent of ADHD risk is attributable to genetic factors.

Importantly, no single gene causes someone to develop ADHD. Instead, it's the combination of many genes that contributes to the unique, inherited vulnerability for ADHD.[1] We can state with confidence that ADHD depends on biological, not social, circumstances. But high heritability doesn't mean that everyone with a certain genetic predisposition will develop full symptoms of ADHD. It does not mean that environmental and social factors are unimportant. However, heritable conditions will, by default, create families where several individuals may struggle with similar difficulties. This may easily give rise to vulnerable family systems. Thus, many parents of children with ADHD will have difficulties of their own to deal with, while simultaneously trying to support and shape the best possible situation for their children.

There are many graphic instances of the interplay between genes and the environment in which they operate. According to one much publicized study, our genetic makeup may determine how we react to adverse events or trauma. Put simply, some of us are born with a genetic vulnerability to be more adversely affected in the instance of trauma, neglect, or abuse.[2]

The insight that it isn't a case of nature *or* nurture but rather of our genes *in* a specific environment may also explain why not all babies born in deprived environments develop difficulties. We speak sometimes of 'the resilient dandelions', referring usually to children who manage surprisingly well despite a deprived and sometimes abusive home environment and who, unlike their parents or siblings, don't develop mental health problems.

The theory behind this is that some individuals have innate resistance, or resilience, to the impact of their childhood environment, be it deprived, normal, or exceptionally favourable. On the other hand, there are other individuals whom we might call 'the sensitive orchids' who have an innate vulnerability, making them particularly exposed to difficult childhood circumstances and a deprived upbringing.

If these orchid-children grow up in an observant, respectful, and responsive environment, they often grow into fully functional, happy adults. The sensitive orchids, though, often struggle even under 'normal' circumstances. Just like orchid flowers, they need very special care and attention if they are to come into bloom.

Women with ADHD often describe feeling sensitive and misunderstood. Unfortunately, children with ADHD are rarely given a chance to grow up in exceptionally supportive environments. Not because their parents don't want or seek to give them the best start in life – in fact, these parents are often particularly insightful. But rather, since a susceptibility to ADHD is frequently inherited, many parents of children with ADHD, despite their will and insight, can't always create a protective environment for themselves and their children. Regardless, it's still important that others understand that ADHD is not a result of bad parenting but can affect the parents as well as the children with ADHD. Just like all children with disabilities, those with ADHD need understanding and support. Therefore, to help the child, we may need to support the entire vulnerable family system on several levels.

Being a parent with ADHD

Sometimes I talk to young women with ADHD who say they do not want their own children. This often isn't due to a lack of desire for a family, but rather because they don't trust themselves to be responsible for another living being. Also, many women diagnosed with ADHD in adulthood report that they were able to compensate for their difficulties if they only had themselves to take care of, but as soon as children entered the equation things became unmanageable. For lots of women with ADHD, the parental stress is high, and feeling that being a parent is beyond their capacity is common.

You might end up in a situation where the routines you have trusted for years suddenly are no longer adequate, or you might have to put an extraordinary amount of time into organizing simple everyday tasks, tasks that others seem to take in their stride. Perhaps you have started to realize that all your energy goes into just getting through the day. And indeed, few things are more painful and unbearable for a parent than to suspect that you are failing to meet your child's needs. Many mothers with ADHD can experience a constant feeling of failure, along with judgement and negative attention from others.

Families with ADHD often need support and intervention from society. In an ideal world, this would be provided with a sensitivity towards each family's specific needs. Sad to say, many women with ADHD tell us that social and care services do not often deliver respect and understanding. 'ADHD families' rarely make the perfect patients or clients, especially when they fail to keep appointments or act on agreed treatment plans. Often, providers of support and treatment, like me, end up falsely accusing families of not being 'motivated enough' and close their case if they don't show up. When someone self-medicates with alcohol or drugs, they are sometimes advised not to come back until they've tackled their harmful habits. When they are angry and disappointed with their professional care, we might feel that it's more an expression of ingratitude or entitlement.

As previously discussed, the high heritability of ADHD will create exposed and vulnerable family systems, where both children and parents struggle much harder than in others, have more conflicts, and feel more stigmatized by society. Some research suggests that mothers of daughters with ADHD suffer more severe parental strain due to their child's ADHD symptoms.[3] And indeed, as previously discussed, delayed ADHD diagnosis, lower access to treatment once diagnosed, and general societal expectations and prejudice may all play a part in that unfortunate reality.

However, we may also find many ADHD mothers becoming

fantastic advocates for their children. Having themselves been side-lined, misunderstood, and exposed is a great driver in their quest to ensure that their own child doesn't ever have to endure the same treatment.

T, THE TIGER MUM

T has three children and her oldest daughter, C, was diagnosed with ADHD two years ago. Her two younger daughters are very much like their father in personality and abilities; however, C is a carbon copy of a younger T. T would describe C as an anxious daydreamer with a big heart and a vivid imagination. When C did the assessment for ADHD, T realized that she probably also had ADHD. She underwent an assessment and was diagnosed about a year ago.

Preschool and school were hard for C. C didn't want her parents to leave her, her assimilation took forever, and T often left the preschool heavy-hearted and full of worry, drying her tears as she drove off to work. However, according to the staff, C was fine once T left. Eventually, preschool passed without any concern from the staff and teachers. However, during primary school, T began to worry that C was lagging behind.

She was in regular touch with the school but was always reassured. Things were fine – C was well behaved and popular with the staff and the other pupils. T thought that she was probably just an over-anxious first-time mother. She felt that the staff were likely irritated that she was never satisfied with their reassurances that C was 'just like any other eight-year-old'.

But T's memories of her own schooldays were still a little too fresh. She remembered the feeling of not understanding how she would complete schoolwork, spending far too much time idle and then suddenly realizing she'd been staring out of the window during the lesson. She remembered the shame of hearing her classmates giggle when she missed the unspoken rules of a game or said the wrong thing, being embarrassed by her parents, and the break out of laughter when she walked out to the pool having forgotten to put on her swimsuit. At that time, she had nowhere to turn for advice or comfort. T lived her entire childhood and half her adult life feeling different from everyone else. But this feeling of 'difference-ness' had no name and she concluded she was defective somehow.

As the mother of a wonderful little girl so painfully like herself, T couldn't stop worrying that C was having similar school experiences. When C realized that her parents would insist on her going to school every day, she began to complain of stomach pain and headaches. She rarely brought home friends. When T suggested an ADHD assessment, the school was puzzled as they felt that C was neither different nor struggling.

T tried to shake off the feeling that she was an annoying parent and carried on regardless. Unfortunately, the situation deteriorated, and the school thought T was looking for problems that didn't exist, questioning their competence. For T this was a nightmare, and she feared that the now-fraught relationship with the school management would affect C. Meanwhile, the school attributed C's reluctance to go to school to T's over-protective, controlling manner.

The downslide was reversed when C changed class

as she entered middle school. Her new teacher was knowledgeable about and deeply interested in neurodevelopmental disorders such as ADHD, ADD, and autism. For T, this was a decisive factor in daring to release her grip on C and let her find her own way in keeping with her unique strengths and vulnerabilities.

'Just because I think that she's a mini copy of me doesn't mean that my experience is her truth and future. But when you worry about your child and recognize your own failures, it's easy to interpret it in the worst possible way. As a society, we have learned an incredible amount about girls and ADHD since I was C's age 30 years ago. Teachers and school staff are so much better informed today and I'm grateful that C doesn't have to take the same journey as I did.'

The detestable 'life puzzle'

The 'life puzzle' is a hackneyed term that can mean different things to different people. It's often used to describe the stress adults, and in particular parents, can suffer when the work-life balance seems unmanageable. The term becomes problematic, however, if it intimates that everyone struggles equally hard to juggle studies or work and social life, family, children, and ageing parents. In my experience, this is far from the case when it comes to women living with ADHD. Even though the term 'life puzzle' is intended to create a collective feeling of comfort, I rather feel that comparing ourselves to others, without adjusting for our unique prerequisites, often exacerbates feelings of failure and despair.

Women in families where a child is affected by ADHD will tell us that they have many more conflicts, not only between children and parents but also between the parents themselves.

The children have worse diets, get less exercise, and sit more often passively in front of various screens. Does this seem familiar? In addition to all the excessive strain, ADHD families often have to put up with busybodies wagging their fingers and saying, 'It's not so strange that those kids are so unruly and naughty – their parents just let them eat junk food and sit in front of YouTube.'

Russell Barkley, one of the world's most renowned and experienced ADHD researchers, years ago found that when children with ADHD are given the correct diagnosis and treatment, their parents feel better, relate better to each other, and function better.[4] Thus, with proper treatment for the child, the parents become better parents. These results have been repeated and replicated in many subsequent studies following Professor Barkley's important work. Other research groups have confirmed the considerable strain under which families of an ADHD-affected child live.[5] However, this important message hasn't been disseminated or done away with old, flawed truths about childhood ADHD symptoms and the psychosocial family environment – a child's ADHD symptoms are not caused by poor parenting. Furthermore, the fact that children in families where someone has ADHD tend to eat less healthily, exercise less, and have more screen time is often caused by a completely different life puzzle.

In conclusion, ADHD is not caused by sugar, video violence, mobile phones, computer screens, or junk food. At the root of the problem lies a biological disability.

Affection – loving someone with ADHD

Living with ADHD can often leave you with feelings of being misunderstood, that you get misguided advice, or that others place impossible demands on you. All this may well be true. But it's not uncomplicated to love and live with someone who in one moment is a fizzing sparkler and the next a burnt-out tangle of steel wire.

As a parent, partner, or child of someone with ADHD, it simplifies things if you understand what you're struggling with or against. This does *not* mean that you should accept being pushed around, steamrollered, oppressed, or flattened by the fluctuating energy levels and emotional swings of your loved one. To avoid being dragged down into someone else's disability, you need a basic understanding of what ADHD can entail, beyond the hyperactivity, impulsivity, or distractedness.

This lies at the heart of many of the interventions offered after someone receives an ADHD diagnosis. There are groups for adults with ADHD that welcome life partners or other close relatives.

It is a well-known fact that relatives of people with psychiatric disorders and lifelong impairments experience more stress in life and put as much time into supporting and helping their loved one as they might a full-time job. Many family members describe the strain and frustration caused by living with someone affected by ADHD.

Relatives often have the important task of supporting a child or an adult with ADHD in their efforts to find viable strategies for getting through the day. However, a growing number of studies and reports that measure the stress and worry of these families note a lower life quality and higher risk of stress-induced problems such as anxiety and depression. Parents or relatives of a girl or woman with ADHD can also feel shame and guilt for the situation in which their child or partner finds themselves.

Many parents' lives can be marked by anxiety and concern for their child's health, as well as any undesirable behaviour or choices. For a partner, it can be exhausting and challenging to understand and keep up with the sudden swings of motivation, energy, and mood of people affected by ADHD.

Relatives of someone with ADHD have to put energy into helping their loved one, but also take care of themselves, understanding that they're in a role that sometimes seems nothing more than a clean-up. Being able to offload and talk to others can prevent them descending into bitterness and arguments. Sharing experiences with others in similar situations can help immensely.

So, what do we need to know about our partner/loved one/ friend/child with ADHD to help them and ourselves and to save the relationship? First, we may want to consider these truths about ADHD:

- A person is born with or develops ADHD early in life and it is a highly heritable disorder.
- ADHD is not a superpower or a blessing; however, many brave people with ADHD and families of someone with ADHD often are superheroes.
- For people with ADHD, some of the brain's most important structures and functions behave differently compared to those without ADHD.
- Many people with ADHD achieve great things working with their differences rather than struggling against their ADHD.
- ADHD is more than just impaired concentration, hyperactivity, and impulsivity and people with ADHD often have to struggle uphill their whole lives. Acting differently is not an option.
- ADHD is a serious disorder with a good prognosis.

Without the proper support and treatment, people with ADHD are at significant risk of suffering from physical diseases, mental health problems, and harmful alcohol and drug use, as well as criminality, loneliness, alienation, unemployment, divorce, road accidents, and premature death. Consequently, they have a shorter life expectancy than those without ADHD by around ten years.

With these basic facts in mind, it's often easier to make decisions about our own well-being and life choices and to understand what we can and cannot change.

Taking care of ourselves, cultivating our own interests, and staying true to our core values can be the best aid for a partner with ADHD. If we live with someone with ADHD, we need to provide support *and* partnership. The last thing someone with ADHD needs is to feel guilty about letting their problems drag others down with them.

B AND THE BALANCING ACT

B and E met in their first year at university. B still remembers how he fell head over heels for E's charm and intensity.

'She was everything I'd never had in my family and in my previous relationships. She was so spontaneous and unconventional, so full of life, passion, and emotion. So brave and yet so fragile.'

B soon took on the role of E's greatest admirer and protector. He loved the fact that she was so unpredictable but was always a little afraid of losing his place in her life.

'Life with E is never boring. At first, I guess I didn't have much time to think about the position I had been pushed back to. I was too busy trying to keep up with E's pace and piece together the fragments of her when she got herself into trouble, fell out with someone, or just lost her self-confidence or direction in life.'

In more recent years, it became increasingly clear to B, however, that this emotional roller-coaster they were both being tossed around in was taking more of a toll on him than on E.

'It's more like a natural state for E, who can be scintillatingly exalted one second and totally desolate the next. At first, I tried to keep up, to be engaged, support and suggest ways of dealing with everything, glossing over it. But I gradually just got more and more inured to it, in a bad way, I think. I felt burnt out by all the sudden whims and ideas. I found myself almost feeling relieved when E was low and subdued. It gave me time to rest, to recuperate. And I didn't have to fear her heading off on some new escapade.

'I really didn't like this dynamic that had been built into our relationship and I slowly turned into a bitter nay-sayer who didn't feel like doing anything at all any more. And I noticed that I kept falling into the role of the nurturer, but it was so tiring to find that she never seemed to learn from her failures. It wasn't long before I couldn't stand to hear my own voice. I sounded like a broken record: "What did I tell you? You said you'd sort out the kitchen before going to work. But what's got into you? How did you think it'd make me feel?"

'The group therapy we took after E's assessment and

diagnosis was hugely important to me. There were eight couples there, including us, where one in each pair had just been diagnosed with ADHD and the others were people who'd had ADHD in their lives without understanding either their partner or themselves. On the outside, we were very different, but we shared so many experiences and emotions that it got ridiculous at times. The course gave me a chance to share my thoughts and feelings with other partners, and I gained a much better understanding that E often can't do anything about how she behaves. Parallel with E being helped by her new insights, I also got a little restoration. It became clear to us both that we wouldn't be dancing this dance any more.

'I needed to be better at taking care of myself and cultivating my own interests, and E gained new tools for getting her life better ordered and more structured. I was able to let go of the role of fixer, planner, and cleaner. Strangely, E's assessment and ADHD diagnosis were the best things that happened to us. It might not be the first thing you think about when someone in your family gets diagnosed with a lifelong disability, but that's what it was like for us.'

Having a parent with ADHD

The human is an exceptional mammal to the extent that its offspring enter the world so utterly immature. Comparing a human baby with the cub of our mammalian relatives, we find that our species will stay dependent on the care of its progeny for a much longer time.

One reason for our relative helplessness is the complicated and advanced human brain. Everything that needs to fit into our brain would never fit inside the newborn skull – at least if this skull was to pass through a woman's birth canal. Nature had to decide whether to reshape the female skeleton to the detriment of their ability to migrate and move across large areas or flee from predators or enemies, or to adapt the nervous system so that it would continue to develop in pace with the increasing girth of the head with age after birth.

This compromise, however, is not uncomplicated or without risk. The many years it takes our immature brain to reach its full potential leaves us dependent on adults and caregivers who will train us in what's right and wrong and protect us from dangers. It is therefore quite natural for babies to do what they can to obtain the acceptance and protection of parents and adults. For the vast majority, this arrangement works. Most parents do their utmost to be the best possible version of their adult-selves in relation to their children. But what is it like to be a child of a parent who, despite the will and desire for nothing else, is not fully capable of providing the essentials for their child?

It is not only important that we understand what it is like to live with ADHD yourself or have a partner with ADHD, but we must also try to understand what it can be like to be the child of a parent with ADHD. A-M's story below is important and gives us many penny-dropping insights, and tips on how an adult with ADHD, notwithstanding their own difficulties, can be a perfectly good enough parent. And it's a moving example of how it's never too late to have a happy childhood.

A-M AND THE ADHD MOTHER

A-M is not so much like her mother; in fact, she sees more of herself in her father, the parent who has always bestowed security and stability on her life. A-M has always loved her mother though and now, as adults, they have a fulfilling, mutually respectful relationship. But it hasn't always been so, and things were much more complicated when A-M was growing up.

A-M remembers being an anxious child, always seeking the attention and validation of the adults. It was particularly important for her that her mother was happy. She vividly remembers the feelings of insecurity, sometimes bordering on fear, as she waited for her mother to get home from work. What kind of day had she had today? Had someone been horrible to her? Had someone upset her or tired her out? Had it been a tough day, or would her mother come home fizzing with energy and lift her into the air and take her on a spontaneous bike ride to buy ice-cream?

It was never the physical turmoil around her mother that disturbed A-M. It didn't matter so much that she always seemed to be losing her keys, glasses, handbag, and purse, that their house was always messier than her friends', or that her mother sometimes forgot school outings, parent-teacher meetings, or to stock the fridge with A-M's favourite snacks.

As an adult, she understood that much of her anxiety was about never quite knowing, and trying to adapt to, her mother's quickly changing moods. It was difficult to feel more mature and stable than her mother when she was as young as 12. And it was scary when her mother plummeted into poor self-esteem or when she would blame herself or others for her failures. It was even a bit frightening when her mother was in an exuberant mood, when, despite her fast pace and gaiety, A-M would always have a nagging worry that the atmosphere could change as quickly as it had arrived.

As an adult, A-M has been able to discuss all this with her mother. Following a serious depression and burnout, her mother underwent an ADHD assessment. A-M was part of the entire process and contributed important information throughout. Subsequently, A-M and both her parents attended a group course on ADHD for people who had recently been diagnosed with ADHD and their adult children. These meetings and conversations were as valuable to A-M as to both her parents.

A-M says that she wished her mother had received help and support earlier, as maybe it would have made her own childhood easier to enjoy and comprehend. At the same time, A-M is grateful that she is now able to understand and forgive her mother for what she was unable to give her as a child. She knows her mother loves her and did her best given the personal problems that she was wrestling with.

It means a lot that her mother has insight into her problems now and takes responsibility for her part in the life they shared for so many years. It's also healing to see that her mother is a wonderful grandmother to A-M's daughter P, who is so much like her grandmother.

Notes

1   Larsson *et al.*, 2013
2   Klengel & Binder, 2015
3   Bussing *et al.*, 2003; Hallberg *et al.*, 2008
4   Barkley *et al.*, 1992
5   Bauer *et al.*, 2019

Chapter 9

Working Life

For many people, ADHD entails a life with a diminished ability to structure, organize, and prioritize everyday activities. Women with ADHD often devote an incredible amount of energy to getting through the day, often without anyone else realizing how much it takes for them to perform tasks at work that others find simple.

Maybe you do some of those things that many other women with ADHD do to conceal their impairments. Or end up in situations where you bring your work home so you can catch up while others are free. Perhaps you get your assignment submitted in time, but at the cost of not getting enough rest and recuperation. For some, this will trigger a downward spiral that, at worst, ends in total exhaustion – much to the incomprehension of everyone else. 'She has exactly the same things to do as all of us other colleagues. No one makes any extra demands on her.'

In a large-scale study on the effects of ADHD among adult employees in ten different countries, researchers found that ADHD was common – over 3 per cent – and usually undiagnosed in the workplace. Workers with ADHD had more absence and sick leave compared to those without a diagnosis. Hardly surprisingly, they were also more often in treatment for mental problems and substance abuse than adult employees without ADHD.[1]

Studies and reports indicate that much can be gained by ensuring that adults with ADHD obtain the correct diagnosis, explanatory model, and treatment in both their professional and their personal lives. This could also benefit colleagues and employers. Unfortunately, few employers take an interest in this large group of employees, whom they could easily help work so much more efficiently and who, given the right conditions, could be an incredibly valuable resource in the workplace.

F AND THE AIRPORT

A good example of how someone with ADHD can experience their working life is an analogy I have borrowed from F, a young woman with ADD. F tells me that she sees her brain like a major international airport. There's the constant noise of airplanes taking off, landing, and taxiing back and forth. Luggage trucks crossing the runways need to be matched up with the right airplane to make sure the passengers' personal effects don't end up on the wrong continent. Delays, cancellations, and iced-up wings need to be factored in to the constantly changing schedule. But F says that she doesn't have anyone working in the control tower at her airport. In other words, she lacks someone able to manage all the central functions needed to coordinate the extremely complex movements at the airport and avoid life-threatening disasters.

F can describe quite vividly what it's like to live with poor executive functions. The feeling of not being able to rely on information being processed and fed back automatically means that F continuously must put energy into being her own control tower. It's not hard to imagine that this is very energy consuming and draining.

'So,' she says, 'if a plane is two minutes late, it affects everything that day. It changes everything and I have to adjust my entire day so that nothing goes wrong. If a plane is delayed for you others, without ADHD, you can probably just lean back in the comfy airport armchairs and wait for new departure times to flick up on the screens. But I have to drop everything that I'm doing and run out onto the runways to stop all planes and change all schedules and then try to reorganize it all. I just feel the panic rise and I'm just so tired all the time.'

As 'non-ADHD airports' with intact executive functions, we can rest assured that the control tower staff have all eventualities in hand and can automatically make compensatory adjustments. But for F, the energy-draining work doesn't end when she finally manages to restore order at her airport.

Neither can she, unlike people without ADHD, engage the autopilot on the airplanes once they have taken off, but must continue flying them manually, day in, day out. No wonder, then, that she is exhausted by lunchtime, or that she has what she calls 'psycho-collapses' when she gets to work in the morning and the meeting she has prepared for has been pushed back to the afternoon instead.

And neither is it hard to understand that she has no energy for socializing, free-time activities, or doing anything at all other than lying down in a quiet room watching old Netflix series and hoping that she'll be able to rest her overheated brain until everything starts all over again in the morning.

The ADHD and subsequent post-diagnosis interventions that F has received have been a huge help and comfort to her. They can communicate to others that she needs rest and recuperation in a way that people without ADHD don't. This doesn't mean, as she once thought, that she's a person who thrives best on her own and who should avoid social occasions. The times when she has withdrawn too much, her mood and health have plummeted, and she has tended to feel miserable and lonely.

Instead, F has learned not to compare herself with others whose brains are wired differently. She just needs to plan breaks before and after multi-sensory exposed situations. Again, for most people, the brain's super-complex calculations and alternative plans of action come automatically and at a much lower cost, and it can be hard to understand how someone not born with this capacity experiences life and struggles to get through their day. But F's brilliant metaphor gives us a thorough understanding of her everyday challenges.

On the art of daydreaming at the wrong time

It's a well-known fact that people with ADHD find it hard to maintain focus, concentration, and pay attention when required to do so. When tasks are monotonous or not sufficiently stimulating, many with ADHD will lose focus as the brain starts to seek more exciting input that can keep it occupied and awake. One theory is that the ADHD brain has trouble switching between parallel networks involved in performing a task.

These two networks are often called the default mode network – which for simplicity's sake we might regard as the daydreamer brain – and the task positive network or the central executive network, which we can call the problem-solver brain.[2]

We might conceptualize it as the 'screensaver' being activated in the daydreamer brain when we don't need to focus that closely on a task but can let our thoughts wander. However, we also expect our problem-solver network to remain active when we take on tasks that are challenging. In this mode, we need access to our previous experiences of similar situations, our powers of reasoning, and our working memory.

Most people can switch between these networks so efficiently that they're not even aware they're doing it. They simply engage the structures and networks requiring higher mental functions when doing complex tasks and switch over to the daydreamer network when doing routine tasks.

Many with ADHD, however, describe that the wiring between the two networks seems faulty. This may put them in awkward as well as dangerous situations. Someone working with machinery, for example, could easily lose more than a fingertip if engaging their daydreamer brain at a critical moment and it's often extremely difficult to complete a maths problem if the brain's screensaver switches on at the wrong time.

Many girls and women with ADHD describe how frustrating it can be to have their thoughts drift away in situations when they really need to focus and be alert. They feel as if their brain is letting them down when they, in fact, know they can perform if their brain just would start working *with* rather than *against* them. Many will admit how demoralizing it is to be told to 'get a grip' by their unaware colleagues or relatives. To constantly be reminded of how your brain is failing you and the expectations of others eventually breaks even the most confident person.

K AND THE CAREER

K returned to work after a period of maternity leave for her second child, having separated from her first child's father before the child's first birthday. Fortunately, they are still good friends. Less fortunately, her ex lives in another town with his new family, and sorting out the pick-ups, drop-offs, and preschool assimilation for little P along with new work responsibilities and delayed house renovations certainly isn't child's play.

After being diagnosed with ADHD following her first pregnancy, K had a better understanding of herself and her vulnerabilities but felt that she had still a long way to go before she could rely on her new strategies. She didn't know whether to tell her new boss and colleagues about her diagnosis – would it mean greater understanding and support or would it hinder career advancement? Her experiences of how others reacted to her ADHD assessment and diagnosis had so far not been encouraging.

'I was so relieved and full of optimism right after the assessment,' she said. 'It was as if someone really saw me and what I was struggling with for the first time – as if I'd be able to move mountains simply by understanding about myself. I went to this post-diagnosis group course and I really grew from the feeling of not being alone. It was as if I had finally found my tribe. It was so powerful to meet others like me who understood what I was aiming at before I'd even said it out loud.

'And my medication has been a godsend too. But it still felt a little bit that as soon as I left the ADHD clinic I'd walk straight into a wall of prejudice and ignorance. I ended up constantly having to justify and explain my diagnosis and medication in a way that I'd find hard to believe people with diabetes or high blood pressure had to. Those diagnoses aren't visible on the outside either, but few people would suggest that a diabetic should try to adjust their blood glucose through willpower rather than with insulin, would they? Or that it's okay to go about your life with high blood pressure just because it's "natural".'

If K could open up about her ADHD at work, she and her boss could find accommodations and improve her efficiency, thus reducing the risk of her becoming burnt out again. There has been recently a movement in many workplaces to attract a more diverse range of staff. Many employers offer neurodiversity awareness training for staff and have, or are working on, policies to accommodate neurodiverse employees. Courses and trainers are widely available for employers to organize the workplace for their staff. These are positive steps but there is still stigma attached to psychiatric diagnoses and K feels that it may be a risk that any problems or complications will be blamed on her ADHD diagnosis.

While K's workplace and employers are not currently ADHD or neurodiverse aware, many experienced clinicians and researchers would suggest that K might gain something by being open about her disability at work. They would argue that it's not the 'diagnostic label' that causes ADHD discrimination, but rather it's the difficulties and behaviours themselves that stigmatize people with psychiatric diagnoses and disabilities. If this is so, workers don't need to worry about being labelled by their diagnosis, and there is everything to gain from obtaining a diagnosis, swift treatment, and the accommodations at work as well as at home.

Notes

1   de Graaf *et al.*, 2008
2   Sonuga-Barke & Castellanos, 2007

Chapter 10

Performance versus Function

The difference between function and performance

There are many adults with ADHD who perform fantastically well, yet still function terribly. An ADHD assessment always includes an estimation of the degree of the everyday functional impairment. The assessment team normally consists of a psychologist and a psychiatrist but can be supplemented by an occupational therapeutic assessment to map out the different aspects of functional impairment. The aim is always to ascertain how someone functions in their everyday life and the consequences of their ADHD symptoms, and to suggest individualized interventions and accommodations. We are often quick to appreciate how someone excels in a particular area and cite this as an example of success, happiness, and high functionality. This can, however, be quite detached from the person's own experience. Thus, we risk missing the full picture if we only focus on the surface and fail to explore deeper into how their life truly functions.

It can be unfortunate if others fail to see the aspects that function hopelessly poorly in women and girls, and instead just cheer on the bits that operate well. For many with ADHD, performance is often achieved at the cost of other major aspects of life. There are tons of women who are excellent entrepreneurs, artists, or journalists and yet are wholly unable to maintain their health, home, or family.

When others well intentionally encourage and cheer on the performative side of someone, the danger is that other possibly important facets of their life become neglected. Women with ADHD often talk about this very phenomenon – about failing in relationships, and feeling lonely in the midst of accomplishing something. This is probably not unique for women with ADHD, but in my experience, it is a common feature in many of their stories.

ADHD often prevents people from tapping into their full potential. It's not hard to imagine that their energy peters out during the day as they are unable to automate repeatable, manual processes. Colleagues may wonder why a woman with ADHD starts to fade out even before the morning coffee break. And many women with ADHD understand that they have to choose between getting the job done or socializing with friends.

When we just see someone's achievements, it's easy to simplify the situation. In front of us we have a successful woman and top performer. It is easy to be impressed and even envious of that. But in women with ADHD, there is always a flipside to the high achievement, and it is usually far from glamorous.

Hyperfocus, a state in which you experience everything with such ease that you lose a sense of time and space, is something with which many with ADHD are familiar. A feeling of everything proceeding with such ease that you lose your sense of time and space is often regarded as a positive thing.

Still, many women with ADHD report a desire to be able to modulate their energy levels and most would happily swap success for the ability to regulate their internal thermostat in time. The need for recuperation when the opportunity comes too late can drain a person's energy, desire, and capacity, and, in the end, it can become increasingly hard to return to some kind of normality after these 'hyperfocus rushes'. Depression, burnout, and a feeling of constant tiredness and exhaustion are greatly over-represented in women with ADHD. At worst, all talk of ADHD as a superpower can make those with the diagnosis and their families, friends, and colleagues focus too much on one single part of their ADHD without understanding other aspects that may become increasingly problematic.

Encouraging people to take advantage of and exploit their strengths is fundamentally good, but the tools they have for taking care of the less attractive sides of their 'superpower' must not be overlooked. Space for recuperation and rest must be found. To achieve is one thing; to function is quite another.

When examples of successful people with ADHD are raised, one can't help but wonder whether floundering in the wake of these gifted and lionized geniuses (predominantly of male gender, please note) are a host of exhausted and depleted partners, children, colleagues, and friends.

Metacognition – thoughts about one's own thinking

Cognition is, as discussed before, a broad concept that denotes our ability to think and process information, and a collective term for the brain's complex processes and skills. Memory, attention, wakefulness, and executive functions are different parts of our cognition and it is common for both children and adults with ADHD to have difficulties in one or many aspects of their cognitive functions.

Some of these cognitive functions, such as working memory, process speed, and verbal abilities, are quantifiable and can be explained with the aid of neuropsychological tests that are often included in an ADHD assessment. Others, such as emotion regulation and wakefulness, however, are less distinct. We sometimes also talk about metacognition, or our ability to think about our cognitive functions and skills. In other words, the way we think about how we think, emote, and behave. People with strong intellectual faculties often also have strong metacognitive skills. But this might not always be the case. And this may be where things can get additionally complicated for people with ADHD, particularly those with a high IQ.

Metacognition can be divided into two parts: the knowledge of one's cognitive processes and the control of one's thoughts and behaviours on the basis of this knowledge. The gap between the intellectual metacognitive capacities and cognitive functions such as executive functions is sometimes painfully obvious when you live with ADHD.

In addition, there is an overlap between how the brain processes information (i.e. its global executive functions) and intelligence (i.e. its logical, fluid, verbal abilities together with its working memory and processing speed) but one that is not particularly strong in people with ADHD. There are plenty of highly gifted people with ADHD living with a constant rift between what they know they should be able to attain and what they actually accomplish.

If you are gifted and still not performing according to your potential, you will probably feel a permanent sense of inadequacy. A lifelong feeling of having failed socially, academically, and professionally is fertile soil for rock-bottom self-esteem. Neuropsychological testing is an important part of the ADHD assessment. If we chart someone's intellectual capacity, executive skills, and ADHD symptoms during the assessment, and stress the differences between their ADHD and their talents, we have great material to influence future treatment and therapies. For many girls and women with ADHD, it's not until they understand how these complicated processes are tied together that they have a chance to repair their self-image and recover their faith in the future.

Treatment for ADHD is not about making someone 'stick it out' or 'let go'. It's about appreciating and respecting differences on a deeper level, knowing that ADHD is a lifelong disability. Treatment and accommodations can be tailored accordingly.

O AND HER THOUGHTS ABOUT THINKING

O is sitting in the front row watching the movie about her own life as it plays out in front of her. She often says that it's blatantly obvious that her own brain hinders the film's plot development. It's so clear, she says, and yet it seems impossible to change the course of it.

'Sure, it's a pain that everyone else seems to wonder at and condemn my "ADHD behaviour". But the truth is that I'm often even harder on myself. Why don't I just do it right this time? Why don't I just resist the feeling or the impulse, stick it out, and come out the other side for once? How come I keep seeing myself play the lead in a film that ends the same way every time?'

'One of the hardest insights to digest about my ADHD assessment was that it turns out I'm actually pretty clever. According to my psychologist, I have an IQ of 153. Me, who's always tried to cover up my big secret that I must be verging on being intellectually disabled, or mentally retarded, as they used to say. And really, I can't think of that as an absurd or unreasonable conclusion – after all, I've always found it so difficult to make even the simplest things turn out as I want. I'm not really sure what to do with this new information. It's bittersweet in so many ways. All the negative, demeaning, belittling things I have thought and said about myself and my intellect over the years. All the things that in theory seem so obvious and easy that just don't get done. And all the sadness of feeling like the odd one out, not deserving happiness or success. I guess it will be a long way back, but at least I have started on a new movie script now.'

The problems that many gifted people with ADHD describe are probably not primarily a result of good metacognitive abilities or being intellectually strong. Rather, it has more to do with the underlying cognitive skills being so uneven and so unmatched. The combination of strong intellectual capacity and diminished executive skills is seldom a real boon for self-esteem and self-confidence.

ADHD and life wisdom

Dilip V. Jeste is a US psychiatrist and neurologist who has combined the ancient content of the mythological Hindu poetry of *Bhagavad Gita* with modern neuroscience to contemplate the concept of wisdom.

Jeste writes about different aspects of what we define as wisdom and, in looking at his ideas about wisdom, we can understand why many people with ADHD do not always consider themselves particularly smart, regardless of their intelligence level.[1]

To begin with, Jeste addresses social skills and openness. This concerns our ability to process the thoughts and opinions of others that may differ from our own. Our traits of empathy, our interest in others, and the extent we take others into account when making decisions are involved as well.

However, it soon becomes much more problematic when Jeste starts pinpointing some of the key features of wisdom that are in stark contrast to how many with ADHD would describe themselves. In Jeste's model, wisdom requires emotional regulation, self-insight, and resolve – that is to say, control over your emotions and how they are expressed.

Problems of self-insight and introspection make it difficult to make decisions based on the best possible knowledge. People with ADHD often find that things go unpredictably wrong and realize that they repeatedly make rash decisions based on too little information. If we accept Jeste's reasoning about wisdom, it's not hard to see that truly intelligent and gifted people with ADHD still can feel very stupid.

With the right support and effective strategies, these difficulties can be managed and compensated for, provided they are properly understood. This is probably why we are surrounded by so many super-smart *and* wise people with ADHD.

Ä AND THE BROODY BRAIN

Ä wanted to talk about her inability to make even the most insignificant decisions and her tendency to dwell over things that have gone wrong or situations where she has made bad choices.

'It's strange, actually. I'm so forgetful and distracted, yet I seem to have the memory of an elephant when it comes to things I'd like nothing more than to forget. I can still, at the age of 38, dwell on stupid things I said to someone at school or did at work a decade ago. I can get totally stuck in my own thought loops about what I did wrong, what I should've done, and why I didn't just do it. These are usually situations in which I feel that I've made a fool of myself.

'I'm tormented by all this brooding. I know that what's been done can't be undone and the rational part of my brain tells me that others likely forgot about it ages ago. If, that is, they even noticed it in the first place.

'When I did my ADHD assessment, my psychologist told me that it's quite common for people with ADHD to dwell on things. She said that one of the consequences of living a life of impulsivity, attention deficits, and diminished executive abilities is that decisions are sometimes made too fast with too little or the wrong information. The penny dropped for me then – me, who has screwed up so many times – that brooding might be a dysfunctional defence mechanism for not making so many painful mistakes.

'The principle then would be that the dwelling and

ruminating would stop me from doing the wrong thing and shaming myself. But instead of preventing it, the brooding created yet another obstacle blocking my perception of social signals. So, what was conceived as a form of protection has become an endless ping-pong match inside my head that just causes me more suffering and failure.

'The insights and support I've had since my ADHD diagnosis have been a huge help, not least for my tendency to dwell on things. However, the first medication I got started on made me even more rigid in my thinking and I got bogged down even more in my own thoughts. During this period, I found it even harder than before the medication to think flexibly and openly. The second medication I tried didn't have that downside and has been really helpful.

'It's not as if a pill per se helps to erase my tendency to ruminate, but it has helped me to accept advice and find better strategies. My brooding is no longer a daily cause of suffering or hindrance.

'I had several CBT treatments for this before my ADHD diagnosis, but they never had any lasting effect and I always just fell into the same rumination rut within a few weeks. It's great that it seems to work now, that the same advice and information are actually having an impact on me. It appears as if it wasn't more facts that needed adding but rather that I had to understand on a deeper level why my brain so easily got hung up on things. The insight into how my ADHD brain works has enabled me to let go of certain thought loops and put up with not returning all those ping-pong serves fired at me by my opponent – my ADHD-broody brain.'

Notes

1   University of Chicago, 2020

Chapter 11

The Years Pass, the ADHD Lasts

ADHD and the life of loneliness

Most studies agree that approximately 5–7 per cent of all children and adolescents meet the criteria for an ADHD diagnosis. But how many older people with ADHD do you know? Often these people have had their difficulties explained away by others as just being hopeless or lazy. But today, in fact, many older people, often because they can see their own difficulties reflected in their children or grandchildren, begin to think about their own life battles and start to re-evaluate their own life patterns.

They will often describe a life with headwinds, but also an uncontrollable desire to try just one more time, often with a liberating self-distance and pragmatism.

Many will say that they finally understand why their own childhood was so chaotic and full of conflicts. That insight alone can be very healing, even if it comes one or two generations too late. Many will tell of a life bordered by periods of exhaustion, of break-ups from work and relationships, of an incomprehensible and judgemental environment, and of failing self-esteem. Many will also have found strategies that have worked for them at times, when work, family, and perhaps a supportive partner have created structure and routines. But there are also many who talk about how these frameworks and routines collapse during periods of change, when working life changes, or when they lose a beloved life partner who, without others knowing, has created absolutely crucial support and structure.

It is not that long ago that it was still very unusual to assess and diagnose adults with ADHD. Despite rapidly growing research of adult ADHD, the number of studies examining how ADHD affects the lives of middle-aged and over-50 adults is still limited. All studies agree that ADHD is an important and impairing disorder, even in middle-aged and older adults.[1] However, in reality, the vast majority of older adults living with ADHD do not have a formal diagnosis.

At present, it's thus quite unusual for women over the age of 65 to be diagnosed with ADHD. Consequently, a substantial amount of middle-aged and older women will live their lives struggling with difficulties due to ADHD without ever getting the right support and treatment.

We have much to gain from a better understanding of how the neuropsychiatric diagnoses manifest during different stages of life. Women with ADHD are at a greater risk not only of comorbidities but also of lifestyle-related diseases, such as obesity, cardiovascular disease, gastrointestinal disorders, and pain.[2] So even if these women have not had a formal ADHD diagnosis, they are often already patients within the healthcare system, receiving medical treatment for other conditions.

We can prevent many of the adverse health consequences by

taking a generational and life-course perspective on ADHD. The vast majority of middle-aged and older women with ADHD have lived their entire lives without understanding patterns of repeated impairments and failures. Older women with ADHD describe, just like younger women, how they feel different and rejected on account of their personality. But they also report that after receiving a diagnosis, they have found it easier to accept themselves and find effective strategies for dealing with their difficulties, even later in life.[3]

ADHD, dementia, or both?

Historically, ADHD has been considered a diagnosis mainly reserved for the young. Consequently, there is little research on the risk of age-related disorders, such as dementia. However, since we now know that ADHD often persists into adulthood, there is an increase in interest in more long-term presentations and consequences.

Differentiating between ADHD and age-related neurodegenerative conditions may be tricky, especially since some of the mental impairments that characterize ADHD – such as inattentiveness, forgetfulness, reduced mental stamina, and difficulties organizing or multitasking – also resemble early signs of dementia in the elderly. Furthermore, psychiatric symptoms, such as insomnia, depression, and anxiety, can be common in dementia and prevalent in adults with ADHD. This can interfere with our understanding of the root cause of the symptoms we see in an elderly person seeking clinical attention for their perceived loss of memory and everyday functionality.

We know too little at present to be able to say exactly why, but having ADHD correlates with an increased risk of dementia. Current evidence leads us to believe it is probably not the ADHD but rather that the common risk factors for dementia such as obesity, smoking, and potentially harmful alcohol consumption are more common in people with ADHD.[4] Researchers are currently investigating whether someone has a higher risk of developing dementia due to the stress that ADHD itself exerts on an ageing nervous system.

After a physical assessment that carefully rules out other underlying causes, a diagnosis of dementia can, in many cases, be dismissed. For women with ADHD, we will instead find that the problems for which she seeks help have been present in different presentations her whole life.

There are currently no evidence-based guidelines for the pharmacological treatment of ADHD in people over 65, largely because this age group has been excluded from studies in drug efficacy and safety. In clinical practice, this boils down to a risk-benefit assessment weighing the severity of the ADHD symptoms, the predicted benefit of the medication, and the individual risk factors of medication versus the consequences of untreated ADHD.

Importantly, for young as well as older women, it's never too late to start creating new, healthier habits. We can, given the right circumstances, change and influence all the lifestyle-related risk factors associated with ADHD.

Ö AND THE WISH TO BE PUT TO SLEEP

Ö was 72 years old when she arrived at my practice for an ADHD assessment. She was tired and lonely and described a life fraught with issues for which she wanted an understanding.

'I've always had this kind of internal itch. When I was a little girl, I never wanted to sleep. I was loud, noisy, and mouthy and sat more outside the classroom than in it, as I remember. But I still felt that I was popular, and think I was fairly accepted by adults and teachers, even though I was pretty unusual for being a girl, especially back in those days. But since junior school, my life has been controlled by a need to scratch this constant itch. I've never been able to sleep, and for a while when I was little, I was even admitted to a psychiatric institution because my mother was totally exhausted, and the doctors didn't know how to put a stop to me and my energy. I was given lots of heavy medication and sedatives and at times during my childhood I think they almost kept me drugged up because they didn't know what was wrong with me.

'In my teenage years, I kept myself occupied. I lived fast and wild, went to a lot of parties, dropped in and out of studies, travelled, rode my motorbike – well, anything that could make me feel something. Or rather, that could stop me feeling so much. I've always had a constant inner drive that doesn't seem to have any direction. I just want to do something, get things done, keep moving. I've been a heavy drinker and in and out of jobs and brief relationships. My great sorrow is my three kids who have three different dads and who I've never been able to form any attachment to. They've grown up, looked after by relatives, their fathers, and the social services, and today they don't want to know me. I suppose I'll never get to know my grandkids. I've run and run through life. Literally, too. I've jumped from one way of trying to scratch this itch to another. For a time, I took to jogging, until my knees and one hip gave up on me. So, I turned to booze and pills, but strangely enough I also always had that kind of internal handbrake when things went too far. So, I've always made sure not to get hooked up for too long on the same substance, medication, or solution. I'm in Alcoholics Anonymous and Narcotics Anonymous and in lots of other support groups. It helps for some things, but not for the itch. I've never felt that I don't want to live. I just feel that I can't live like this. My body and soul have had it. They are worn out. I just want you to put me to sleep.'

Notes

1 Kooij *et al.*, 2016; Goodman *et al.*, 2016; Surman & Goodman, 2017; Dobrosavljevic *et al.*, 2020; Guldberg-Kjär *et al.*, 2013
2 Instanes *et al.*, 2018
3 Henry & Jones, 2011
4 Callahan *et al.*, 2017

Chapter 12

Personal and Professional Treatment

Many people experience relief and hope for the future when getting their ADHD diagnosis. At the very least, this is the start of a new life with new insight and new tools. Unfortunately, however, not everyone is given the personal treatment and support they had hoped for.

B-M AND HOW SHE WAS TREATED

B-M had just undergone an assessment and received her ADHD diagnosis. She was shaken yet relieved and a little sad about all the years she had lost living with the wrong explanatory model and toolbox.

'During the feedback, my psychologist told me that I should work out three different "information packages" about my ADHD that I could prepare to present to different people around me. It's been incredibly valuable and given me the opportunity to own my story, and face everything that I didn't know would come. Comments such as, "A smart woman like you can't have ADHD" or, "Well, everyone's got a touch of ADHD these days. If I went to a psychologist, I bet I'd get diagnosed too" are common. I'd forever find myself having distressing discussions, going on the defensive, getting angry and upset when people would toss stupid comments like that around. I just wanted to scream, "You have to have a disability! And as long as ignorance and tactlessness aren't formal disabling diagnoses, you've got nothing to worry about!" But with my different sized "information packages" I'm prepared now, and don't get all emotional like that. It's better for me, and better for everyone else too.'

Multimodal treatment

Multimodal treatment is the evidence-based treatment recommended for children and adults diagnosed with ADHD. The term multimodal refers to having access to three different types – modalities – of treatment: psychoeducation (education about and knowledge of ADHD), cognitive aids (everyday support and assistive technology), and medication.[1]

Psychoeducation

An important part of segueing towards improved everyday function and well-being following an ADHD diagnosis is learning more about what ADHD is and what it entails for each individual person. This support intervention is called psychoeducation and involves different forms of ADHD education with practical advice on how to handle and solve practical everyday problems.

This kind of intervention can be provided in the form of parental support programmes or group meetings for adults and accompanying relatives. The aim is to improve their knowledge of and provide information about treatment options and societal support, and to help them find relevant and fact-checked information, such as articles, booklets, internet links, and interest groups.

Cognitive aids – support and aids for memory and everyday functionality

Children and adults with ADHD often require concrete support to structure their lives, cope with everyday routines, remember tasks, and keep appointments. These cognitive aids are designed to compensate for cognitive and executive difficulties, providing help with planning the day, remembering to get started on things, arriving on time, taking breaks, and improving sleep quality.

This can involve everything from practical and relatively simple low-tech solutions, such as clocks, reminders, or a weight blanket, to more advanced, high-tech digital aids to remind you to take your medication or help you estimate how long it takes to get from one activity or meeting to another.

Medication

The aim of medication is to mitigate ADHD-related symptoms, enhance everyday function, improve life quality, and prevent common consequences of ADHD, such as low self-esteem and psychiatric and physiological morbidity.

Drugs in themselves rarely bring order to patients' lives. They don't sit down and do your homework, nor do they order your life in an Excel spreadsheet. Drugs can be seen more as an important means of support for getting your life to work as you need to, like a lifejacket. You still have to swim, but it's easier if you don't keep sinking and choking on water.

Lifestyle factors that can improve ADHD

Regular exercise is important for us all. Interestingly, science also clearly shows that physical activity is particularly beneficial to you if you have ADHD. Many studies point towards the same conclusion: exercise can have a positive influence on brain maturation, development, and daily function.

During physical activity that raises our pulse and respiratory rate over a prolonged, uninterrupted period of time, certain hormones and substances are released in our blood stream. We find that exercise, through mechanisms enhanced by these endogenous substances, can have a similar, albeit not as powerful effect as drugs on core ADHD symptoms. What's more, it seems as if drugs and physical activity are mutually enhancing in their efficacy.

The nature of the exercise doesn't appear to matter, so the old saying 'the best exercise is the exercise that gets done' very much applies to ADHD. Brief or temporary exercise is also good, but what seems to be particularly beneficial is regular routines and long-term, repeated physical activity. Unfortunately, many with ADHD report that such regularity is difficult to achieve, even though they know it would be good for them.

It's not just the ability to concentrate, take informed decisions, or change strategy that is improved by exercise and physical activity. Apart from enhancing physical fitness and lowering the risk of other lifestyle and ADHD-related problems such as obesity, cardiovascular disease, and dementia, exercise also reduces the risk of psychiatric comorbidities. Anxiety, depression, and insomnia are common conditions that cause considerable suffering in many people with ADHD, and all can be improved and alleviated with regular physical activity. For those interested in the small but growing field of research on ADHD and exercise the current knowledge is summed up well in a recent review article.[2]

Pharmacological treatment

The psychiatrist has an important, albeit often slightly smaller, role in the neuropsychiatric assessment that in some cases will result in an ADHD diagnosis. They ensure that any physical or mental comorbidities are identified and described and that the symptoms someone describes and presents with are not better attributed to some other psychiatric or physiological condition.

The psychiatrist also examines whether any medical conditions in the diagnosed patient would mean that certain medications are contraindicated or should be used with caution. The physician then will be responsible for initiating and following up the pharmacological treatment agreed on.

The history behind ADHD medication

Much of what we know about ADHD stems from insights into the effects that certain chemical substances (i.e. central stimulant compounds) have on the core symptoms associated with ADHD. By a lucky coincidence, at the end of the 1930s the US physician Charles Bradley discovered that amphetamine-based drugs helped to improve the hyperactivity, social skills, and scholastic results of externalizing children with learning difficulties. This discovery was almost forgotten until methylphenidate was introduced in the US in 1954. Methylphenidate was, however, first recommended for abnormal fatigue, depression, weakness during convalescence, concentration deficiencies, and memory disorders in adults but was later also approved for ADHD in both children and adults. A few years later, during the 1960s, another class of central stimulants was discovered and introduced, the dexamphetamines. Since then, these two major classes of ADHD drugs have evolved to include instant-release, moderate-release, and long-acting preparations to better suit an individual treatment regimen.[4]

Modern ADHD treatment

There are today five different substances from three different classes of drugs that are approved for the treatment of ADHD: methylphenidate, dexamphetamine, and lisdexamphetamine from the central stimulants; atomoxetine from the antidepressants; and guanfacine from the antiadrenergic agents.

There is a great deal of empirical evidence and clinical experience showing that drugs used to treat ADHD are effective and safe.[5] Few pharmacological compounds have been more extensively studied than those for ADHD, very much on account of them being used in children and adolescents. According to most studies, about 70 per cent of those who are prescribed ADHD medication will experience alleviation from the core symptoms of ADHD. Serious adverse reactions are rare and most of the common side-effects are transitory or can be managed by changing between labels and compounds or by adjusting the dose.

Many studies are limited, however, by what is practically and financially feasible to explore. For example, it is impossible, at least by the methodologies and designs used today, to follow individuals randomly assigned to different treatment alternatives over many years. Although there are plenty of well-conducted longitudinal follow-ups of ADHD treatments that unanimously describe beneficial effects without serious or delayed side-effects, this makes it harder to speak with any certainty about the long-term effects or to generalize this to groups that have not been studied.

However, no ADHD treatment exists in a vacuum. Much of what needs to be changed to improve daily function is based on the other two modalities of the evidence-based ADHD treatment: psychoeducation and cognitive aids.

For many patients, however, a drug treatment will be crucial for the other interventions to succeed. How you react to a certain drug will ultimately be a very personal experience, but among adults it's relatively rare for someone to find just the right drug and dose the first time round. Often, treatment begins with the patient, family, and treatment team working closely together to hammer out an individual treatment strategy, optimizing doses for the optimal symptom control.

Once the right drug and dose have been tailored and once there are no unacceptable adverse reactions or risk factors, the work to find new individual strategies can begin.

L AND HER ADHD DRUGS

'I was 20 the first time I tried an ADHD drug. I'd been quite reluctant for a long time and a little scared of these medicines. You read so much about all this, and many people seem to think they're unnecessary. Some even say that they can be dangerous to your health. And I felt a resistance towards identifying myself as someone who takes a pill to function properly. It felt a little bit defeatist, in fact.

'I can't say that my initial experiences of it were that good. I'd read about people who felt that everything just fell into place, and they suddenly got their life together from the very first dose. It wasn't like that for me. I had to spend a long time testing different drugs and doses. There were side-effects and anxiety and a whole lot of meetings with my doctor. I didn't know what to expect, how it would feel, whether the side-effects would pass, and if I was taking the right dose.

'In the end, we worked out a strategy and dosing that worked for me. Naturally, it's not ideal to have to take medicine in order to get through the day. But personally, for me, it's worth it. It was only when I got diagnosed and tested my way to the right medication that I understood once and for all that not everyone struggles like this! It was a weird insight but also a huge relief to realize that the whole of humanity doesn't actually live this kind of difficult life.'

Are we drugging our patients?

It's not hard to appreciate the anguish parents can feel when having to make the decision to medicate their child for something that they feel is part of his or her personality. As I have said, ADHD is not a disorder that we can cure but rather a way of functioning, what we refer to as a 'functional disability' or 'functional variation'.

Moreover, the drugs often used for ADHD are central stimulants and are similar, if not identical, in their chemical composition to certain drugs that can cause addiction if abused. It might also seem rather paradoxical to use stimulant medication for a diagnosis that is often characterized by hyperactivity and an inability to wind down. But the logic is obvious when we understand the underlying causes of the hyperactivity and restlessness that many people with ADHD report.

As described earlier (Chapter 2 on the brain), it is the under-functioning of the parts of the brain involved in wakefulness and attention that causes many of the problems associated with ADHD. In a sense, we could say that people with ADHD struggle to keep their brain awake by ensuring a constant flow of novel input. So, drugs that increase the signalling activity in certain parts of the brain by boosting or stabilizing dopamine and norepinephrine levels can make people feel calmer, more composed, and more steadily focused on the tasks facing them.

How do we know if we're doing the right thing? Is there any risk or flipside in deciding to medicate for ADHD? These are, and should always be, questions that parents of children with ADHD, adults with ADHD, and prescribing physicians should ask themselves before deciding to initiate treatment. All medical decisions must always draw on the best available knowledge for what may be most effective and suitable for the unique girl or woman in question.

Fortunately, as mentioned above, ADHD drugs are among the most studied medicines we have, largely due to their use for treating children during their physical and mental development. Unfortunately, as also mentioned repeatedly in this book, the majority of studies have been done on boys and men. Nevertheless, we still know a great deal about ADHD drugs today, and we know them to be efficacious and safe if taken in the correct way and in compliance with the instructions of an experienced physician. For some reason, yet to be discovered, girls more seldom get access to medication, even though ADHD drugs are proven to be at least as effective for them as for the boys.

A common concern voiced by adults and parents is whether there are any risks associated with ADHD drugs. Many wonder whether there are risks of getting addicted or if we 'make a child's brain more susceptible to harmful drug use later in life'. The answer to these relevant questions has become increasingly apparent to us over the past few years, and after numerous independent studies and current understanding; the answer is NO.

As we have seen, children and adults with ADHD are, for whatever reason, more likely to fall into harmful use and dependency than their peers without ADHD.[6] But the vast majority of published research papers indicate that early diagnosis and the correct drug regimen will have a solid, protective effect against future substance use problems.[7] Even though it's important to discuss the possible risks of medicating, one might wonder *why* we so rarely discuss the risks of not medicating, because the science behind this question is really gloomy and worrisome.

That said, central stimulants for treating ADHD can be used for non-medical reasons and, in worst-case scenarios, abused. This particularly applies to fast-acting or direct-acting central stimulant medications. All substances able to trigger a burst of brain dopamine levels also have the potential to be taken recreationally – that is, for changing one's mental state or 'getting high'. It is for this reason that central stimulants are scheduled drugs – that is, classed as narcotics.

If short-acting ADHD drugs are not taken as prescribed, taken for the wrong reason, or in higher doses than intended, there is a real danger of harmful consequences, such as addiction. Clear treatment guidelines and prescription and follow-up procedures help us to reduce the risk of people ending up with these kinds of problem.

Notes

1   Faraone *et al.*, 2021
2   Christiansen *et al.*, 2019
3   Leahy, 2017
4   Leahy, 2017
5   Caye *et al.*, 2019
6   Chang *et al.*, 2012; Charach *et al.*, 2011
7   Chang *et al.*, 2014

In Closing...

Why did I think that a book specifically about ADHD in women was necessary? Isn't the suffering and pain caused by this lifelong impairment the same for both sexes? Aren't the accounts of alienation, shame, stigma, and failures always extremely personal and individual, untethered to gender and cultural context? The answer to these questions is of course both yes and no.

Diagnoses such as ADHD – which ultimately are descriptions of different (sometimes extreme) ways of functioning, different behaviours, and, to some extent, personality traits that we all share to one degree or another – will always need to be placed in the context of the individual. In other words, there are huge individual differences among those living with ADHD, and an ADHD diagnosis never exists in a vacuum.

ADHD is diagnosed more often today than, say, 30 years ago. It is widely discussed in the media in terms of 'diagnostic inflation' and the loudest and most critical voices are commonly people with limited personal experiences, journalists, and other professional pundits. For those of us engaged in scientific research and who meet people who have lived a whole life in a headwind, such talk verges on being if not grossly offensive then at least a serious and deeply ignorant invalidation of decades of advanced, high-quality research.

It's true that ADHD can be over-diagnosed. It happens, just as it does with all other diagnoses, when we don't have an exact underlying cause or exact ways to measure objectively. Careless and arbitrary diagnosing is always serious and wrong, and it's always the ADHD patient who suffers the greatest risks following diagnostic slips. Deeming someone to have ADHD when their problems may fit more appropriately into another explanatory model or diagnosis will delay effective treatment and cause unnecessary suffering. One of the greatest hazards of over-diagnosis is diluting the ADHD diagnosis itself.

Girls and women with ADHD already deal with countless prejudices about themselves and their diagnosis. And perhaps most seriously of all, ADHD is still under-diagnosed in girls and women. Outdated and inverted causality claims, such as ADHD being the outcome of a poor upbringing or over-protective/absent parents, trauma, or a reluctance to 'get one's act together', prevent many people from obtaining a viable and credible explanatory model for their lifelong impairments.

The right diagnosis and explanation is often invaluable and it may make all the difference when the pieces fall into place and someone understands why they have 'behaved' so awkwardly their entire life, why they have constantly ended up in the same rut, and why 'good' advice of others and interventions of healthcare professionals have failed. There are many girls and women who, in receiving this controversial diagnosis, have been able to bring about change, access self-care tools, and do so based on their own needs and priorities.

Many women with ADHD will try, start again, and try a little harder. But eventually, when their families, friends, and colleagues, despite repeated explanations and promises, feel that nothing's changing, the explanations turn into hollow excuses and the belief in their own abilities wanes.

Growing up with difficulties regulating your own energy levels, be it a matter of physical hyperactivity, impulsivity, or emotional instability, is a challenge for girls and women as well as their parents, partners, and friends. Often, they need support and security to have the energy and courage to keep struggling and trying, despite the occasional setbacks.

One major theme of this book has been why we have found it so hard to identify girls and women with ADHD and to then provide them with the proper help and support. But what about the future? Will others read this book in 20 years' time and be horrified by how little was known about ADHD in girls and women, and how poorly they were treated? I hope so.

Thanks

This book would not have been possible without the stories and experiences of my amazing patients. Every day you teach me more about ADHD than I could ever read in a textbook or scientific article. You have recounted, read, commented on, and made this book what it is – a support for others who have or have had a life similar to yours. I thank you from the bottom of my heart.

I'd also like to thank all my close friends and colleagues for their honest, wise, and engaged feedback. This book was a collaborative effort, and I thank you all for taking the time to help me through the writing process.

I'd like to give special mention to the following:

Adam Kayser, thank you from the bottom of my heart. Translation from Swedish would not have been possible without your generous donation. I really hope your friends enjoy the English translation.

My reliable and knowledgeable publishers, Ingrid Ericson Sweden, Bjarke Larsen Denmark, Tauno Vahter Estonia, Andy Lim and Professor Bahn Korea, and Sean Townsend (UK/USA/

Australia and New Zealand). It's such a pleasure to work with people who are so sharp, quick, insightful, and flexible.

Professor Markus Heilig, friend, fact-checker and tireless spokesman of the perspectives and rights of our patients.

Professor Henrik Larsson, international authority on ADHD research, and my PhD supervisor back in the day, who has made sure that Sweden contributes to modern, evidence-based ADHD knowledge.

Lena Brandt, friend, statistician, and scholar – thank you for everything, from factorial calculations to grammatical supervision.

Agneta Hellström, dear friend and comrade-in-arms. What Agneta doesn't know about ADHD isn't worth knowing. Thanks for so generously sharing your long experience with me.

Elisabeth Fernell, whose years of knowledge about developmental disabilities and *essence* makes her an invaluable sounding board.

Christin Edmark, for inspirational conversations about life with ADHD and for planting the seed of this book.

Sophie Dow, for her determined, tireless, and unselfish quest to disseminate more evidence-based knowledge about the invisible girls.

Petra Krantz Lindgren, Pia Rehn Bergander, and Helena Kopp Kallner for valuable feedback throughout the writing process.

And all the skilled and inspirational colleagues at SMART Psykiatri: you know who you are.

A special thanks to gifted translator and editor Alison Wheather, Shiny Things, for not letting my patients' voices, and mine, get lost in translation.

Finally, Per, Nike, Klara, Hanna, Alexander and Filip, Kim, Mum and Dad. You are my world; I owe everything to you.

Suggested Reading

Barkley, R.A. *ADHD and the Nature of Self-Control.* 2005. New York, NY: Guilford Press. ISBN 978 1 59385 2 313.

Barkley, R.A. *Executive Functions.* 2012. New York, NY: Guilford Press. ISBN 978 1 46250 5 357.

Barkley, R.A. *When an Adult You Love Has ADHD.* 2016. Washington, DC: American Psychological Association. ISBN 978 1 43382 3 084.

Young, S., Adamo, N., Ásgeirsdóttir, B.B. *et al.* Females with ADHD: An expert consensus statement taking a lifespan approach providing guidance for the identification and treatment of attention-deficit/ hyperactivity disorder in girls and women. *BMC Psychiatry,* 2020; 20(1):404.

References

Arcia, E. & Conners, C.K. Gender differences in ADHD? *Journal of Developmental and Behavioral Pediatrics*, 1998; 19(2):77–83.

Arnold, P.D., Ickowicz, A., Chen, S. *et al.* Attention-deficit hyperactivity disorder with and without obsessive-compulsive behaviours: Clinical characteristics, cognitive assessment, and risk factors. *Canadian Journal of Psychiatry*, 2005; 50(1):659–668.

Bale, T.L. & Epperson, C.N. Sex as a biological variable: Who, what, when, why, and how. *Neuropsychopharmacology: official publication of the American College of Neuropsychopharmacology*, 2017; 42(2):386–396.

Barkley, R.A. The relevance of the Still lectures to attention-deficit/ hyperactivity disorder: A commentary. *Journal of Attention Disorders*, 2006; 10(2):137–140.

Barkley, R.A., Anastopoulos, A.D., Guevremont, D.C. *et al.* Adolescents with attention deficit hyperactivity disorder: Mother-adolescent interactions, family beliefs and conflicts, and maternal psychopathology. *Journal of Abnormal Child Psychology*, 1992; 20(3):263–288.

Barkley, R.A. & Fischer, M. Hyperactive child syndrome and estimated life expectancy at young adult follow-up: The role of ADHD persistence and other potential predictors. *Journal of Attention Disorders*, 2019; 23(9):907–923.

Barkley, R.A. & Peters, H. The earliest reference to ADHD in the medical literature? Melchior Adam Weikard's description in 1775 of attention deficit (Mangel der Aufmerksamkeit, Attentio Volubilis). *Journal of Attention Disorders*, 2012; 16(8):623–630.

Bauer, N.S., Ofner, S., Moore, C. *et al.* Assessment of the effects of pediatric attention deficit hyperactivity disorder on family stress and well-being: Development of the IMPACT 1.0 Scale. *Global Pediatric Health*, 2019; 6:2333794X19835645.

Bengtsdotter, H., Lundin, C., Gemzell Danielsson, K. *et al.* Ongoing or previous mental disorders predispose to adverse mood reporting during combined oral contraceptive use. *European Journal of Contraception & Reproductive Health Care*, 2018; 23(1):45–51. .

Biederman, J., Faraone, S.V., Mick, E. *et al.* Clinical correlates of ADHD in females: Findings from a large group of girls ascertained from pediatric and psychiatric referral sources. *Journal of the American Academy of Child and Adolescent Psychiatry*, 1999; 38(8):966–975.

Biederman, J., Petty, C.R., O'Connor, K.B., Hyder, L.L. & Faraone, S.V. Predictors of persistence in girls with attention deficit hyperactivity disorder: Results from an 11-year controlled follow-up study. *Acta Psychiatrica Scandinavica*, 2012; 125(2):147–156.

Bussing, R., Gary, F.A., Mason, D.M. *et al.* Child temperament, ADHD, and caregiver strain: Exploring relationships in an epidemiological sample. *Journal of the American Academy of Child Adolescent Psychiatry*, 2003; 42, 184–192.

Callahan, B.L., Bierstone, D., Stuss, D.T. *et al.* Adult ADHD: Risk factor for dementia or phenotypic mimic? *Frontiers in Aging Neuroscience*, 2017; 9:260.

Castellanos, F.X. & Tannock, R. Neuroscience of attention-deficit/hyperactivity disorder: The search for endophenotypes. *Nature Reviews Neuroscience*, 2002; 3(8):617–628.

Castle, L., Aubert, R.E., Verbrugge, R.R. *et al.* Trends in medication treatment for ADHD. *Journal of Attention Disorders*, 2007; 10(4):335–342.

Caye, A., Swanson, J.M., Coghill, D. & Rohde, L.A. Treatment strategies for ADHD: An evidence-based guide to select optimal treatment. *Molecular Psychiatry*, 2019; 24(3):390–408.

Chang, Z., Lichtenstein, P., Halldner, L. *et al.* Stimulant ADHD medication and risk for substance abuse. *Journal of Child Psychology and Psychiatry, and Allied Disciplines*, 2014; 55(8):878–885.

Chang, Z., Lichtenstein, P. & Larsson, H. The effects of childhood ADHD symptoms on early-onset substance use: A Swedish twin study. *Journal of Abnormal Child Psychology*, 2012; 40(3):425–435.

Charach, A., Yeung, E., Climans, T. & Lillie, E. Childhood attention-deficit/hyperactivity disorder and future substance use disorders: Comparative meta-analyses. *Journal of the American Academy of Child & Adolescent Psychiatry*, 2011; 50(1):9–21.

Christiansen, L., Beck, M.M., Bilenberg, N. *et al.* Effects of exercise on cognitive performance in children and adolescents with ADHD: Potential mechanisms and evidence-based recommendations. *Journal of Clinical Medicine*, 2019; 8(6):841.

Coghill, D.R., Banaschewski, T., Soutullo, C., Cottingham, M.G. & Zuddas, A. Systematic review of quality of life and functional outcomes in randomized placebo-controlled studies of medications for attention-deficit/hyperactivity disorder. *European Child & Adolescent Psychiatry*, 2017; 26(11):1283–1307.

Cortese, S., Moreira-Maia, C.R., St Fleur, D. *et al.* Association between ADHD and obesity: A systematic review and meta-analysis. *The American Journal of Psychiatry*, 2016; 173(1):34–43.

Cortese, S. & Tessari, L. Attention-Deficit/Hyperactivity Disorder (ADHD) and obesity: Update 2016. *Current Psychiatry Reports*, 2017; 19(1):4.

de Graaf, R., Kessler, R.C., Fayyad, J. *et al.* The prevalence and effects of adult attention-deficit/hyperactivity disorder (ADHD) on the performance of workers: Results from the WHO World Mental Health Survey Initiative. *Occupational and Environmental Medicine*, 2008; 65(12):835–842.

Del Campo, N., Chamberlain, S.R., Sahakian, B.J. *et al.* The roles of dopamine and noradrenaline in the pathophysiology and treatment of attention-deficit/hyperactivity disorder. *Biological Psychiatry*, 2011; 69(12):e145–157.

Derks, E.M., Hudziak, J.J. & Boomsma, D.I. Why more boys than girls with ADHD receive treatment: A study of Dutch twins. *Twin Research and Human Genetics*: official journal of the International Society for Twin Studies, 2007; 10(5):765–770.

Dobrosavljevic, M., Solares, C., Cortese, S. *et al.* Prevalence of attention-deficit/hyperactivity disorder in older adults: A systematic review and meta-analysis. *Neuroscience & Biobehavioral Reviews*, 2020; 118:282–289.

Dorani, F., Bijlenga, D., Beekman, A.T.F. *et al.* Prevalence of hormone-related mood disorder symptoms in women with ADHD. *Journal of Psychiatric Research*, 2021; 133:10–15.

Doyle, R. The history of adult attention-deficit/hyperactivity disorder. *Psychiatric Clinics of North America*, 2004; 27(2):203–214.

Dreher, J.C., Schmidt, P.J., Kohn, P. *et al.* Menstrual cycle phase modulates reward-related neural function in women. *Proceedings of the National Academy of Sciences of the United States of America*, 2007; 104(7):2465–2470.

Elkins, I.J., Saunders, G.R.B., Malone, S.M. *et al.* Mediating pathways from childhood ADHD to adolescent tobacco and marijuana problems: Roles of peer impairment, internalizing, adolescent ADHD symptoms, and gender. *Journal of Child Psychology and Psychiatry*, 2018; 59(10):1083–1093.

Faraone, S.V., Asherson, P., Banaschewski, T. *et al.* Attention-deficit/hyperactivity disorder. *Nature Reviews Disease Primers*, 2015; 1:15020.

Faraone, S.V., Banaschewski, T., Coghill, D. *et al.* The World Federation of ADHD International Consensus Statement: 208 Evidence-based conclusions about the disorder. *Neuroscience & Biobehavioral Reviews*, 2021; 128:789–818.

Franke, B., Michelini, G., Asherson, P. *et al*. Live fast, die young? A review on the developmental trajectories of ADHD across the lifespan. *The Journal of the European College of Neuropsychopharmacology*, 2018; 28(10):1059–1088.

Freeman, M.P. ADHD and pregnancy. *American Journal of Psychiatry*, 2014; 171(7):723–728.

Gardner, W., Pajer, K.A., Kelleher, K.J. *et al*. Child sex differences in primary care clinicians' mental health care of children and adolescents. *Archives of Pediatrics and Adolescent Medicine*, 2002; 156(5):454–459.

Gershon, J. A meta-analytic review of gender differences in ADHD. *Journal of Attention Disorders*, 2002; 5(3):143–154.

Gillberg, C. The ESSENCE in child psychiatry: Early symptomatic syndromes eliciting neurodevelopmental clinical examinations. *Research in Developmental Disabilities*, 2010; 31(6):1543–1551.

Gillberg, C., Gillberg, I.C., Rasmussen, P. *et al*. Co-existing disorders in ADHD – implications for diagnosis and intervention. *European Child & Adolescent Psychiatry*, 2004; 13 Suppl 1:80–92.

Gogtay, N., Giedd, J.N., Lusk, L. *et al*. Dynamic mapping of human cortical development during childhood through early adulthood. *Proceedings of the National Academy of Sciences of the United States of America*, 2004; 101(21):8174–8179.

Goodman, D.W., Mitchell, S., Rhodewalt, L. *et al*. Clinical presentation, diagnosis and treatment of Attention-Deficit Hyperactivity Disorder (ADHD) in older adults: A review of the evidence and its implications for clinical care. *Drugs & Aging*, 2016; 33(1):27–36.

Guldberg-Kjär, T., Sehlin, S. & Johansson, B. ADHD symptoms across the lifespan in a population-based Swedish sample aged 65 to 80. *International Psychogeriatrics*, 2013; 25(4):667–675.

Gur, R.C., Richard, J., Calkins, M.E. *et al*. Age group and sex differences in performance on a computerized neurocognitive battery in children age 8–21. *Neuropsychology*, 2012; 26(2) 251–265.

Hallberg, U., Klingberg, G., Reichenberg, K. *et al*. Living at the edge of one's capability: Experiences of parents of teenage daughters diagnosed with ADHD. *International Journal of Qualitative Studies on Health and Well-being*, 2008; 52–58.

Hasson, R. & Fine, J.G. Gender differences among children with ADHD on continuous performance tests: A meta-analytic review. *Journal of Attention Disorders*, 2012; 16(3):190–198.

Hatta, T. & Nagaya, K. Menstrual cycle phase effects on memory and Stroop task performance. *Archives of Sexual Behavior*, 2009; 38(5):821–827.

Heide, M., Huttner, W.B. & Mora-Bermudez, F. Brain organoids as models to study human neocortex development and evolution. *Current Opinion in Cell Biology*, 2018; 55:8–16.

Heilig, M. *Hon, Han Och Hjärnan*. 2018. Natur & Kultur (in Swedish).

Henry, E. & Jones, S.H. Experiences of older adult women diagnosed with attention deficit hyperactivity disorder. *Journal of Women & Aging*, 2011; 23(3):246–262.

Hinshaw, S.P. Preadolescent girls with attention-deficit/hyperactivity disorder: I. Background characteristics, comorbidity, cognitive and social functioning, and parenting practices. *Journal of Consulting and Clinical Psychology*, 2002; 70(5):1086–1098.

Hinshaw, S.P., Owens, E.B., Zalecki, C. *et al*. Prospective follow-up of girls with attention-deficit/hyperactivity disorder into early adulthood: Continuing impairment includes elevated risk for suicide attempts and self-injury. *Journal of Consulting and Clinical Psychology*, 2012; 80(6) 1041–1051.

Hoogman, M., Bralten, J., Hibar, D.P. *et al*. Subcortical brain volume differences in participants with attention deficit hyperactivity disorder in children and adults: A cross-sectional mega-analysis. *Lancet Psychiatry*, 2017; 4(4):310–319. Erratum in: *Lancet Psychiatry*, 2017; 4(6):436.

Hosain, G.M., Berenson, A.B., Tennen, H. *et al*. Attention deficit hyperactivity symptoms and risky sexual behavior in young adult women. *Journal of Women's Health*, 2012; 21(4):463–468.

Ingalhalikar, M., Smith, A., Parker, D. *et al*. Sex differences in the structural connectome of the human brain. *Proceedings of the National Academy of Sciences of the United States of America*, 2014; 111(2):823–828.

Instanes, J.T., Klungsoyr, K., Halmoy, A. *et al*. Adult ADHD and comorbid somatic disease: A systematic literature review. *Journal of Attention Disorders*, 2018; 22(3):203–228.

Jiang, H.Y. *et al*. Maternal and neonatal outcomes after exposure to ADHD medication during pregnancy: A systematic review and meta-analysis. *Pharmacoepidemiology and Drug Safety*, 2019; 28(3):288–295.

Justice, A.J. & de Wit, H. Acute effects of d-amphetamine during the follicular and luteal phases of the menstrual cycle in women. *Psychopharmacology*, 1999; 145(1):67–75.

Justice, A.J. & de Wit, H. Acute effects of estradiol pretreatment on the response to d-amphetamine in women. *Neuroendocrinology*, 2000; 71(1):51–59.

Kaisari, P., Dourish, C.T., Rotshtein, P. *et al*. Associations between core symptoms of Attention Deficit Hyperactivity Disorder and both binge and restrictive eating. *Frontiers in Psychiatry*, 2018; 9:103.

Keltner, N.L. & Taylor, E.W. Messy purse girls: Adult females and ADHD. *Perspectives in Psychiatric Care*, 2002; 38(2):69–72.

Kessler, R.C., Adler, L., Barkley, R. *et al.* The prevalence and correlates of adult ADHD in the United States: Results from the National Comorbidity Survey Replication. *The American Journal of Psychiatry,* 2006; 163(4):716–723.

Klengel, T. & Binder, E.B. Epigenetics of stress-related psychiatric disorders and gene x environment interactions. *Neuron,* 2015; 86(6):1343–1357.

Kok, F.M., Groen, Y., Fuermaier, A.B. & Tucha, O. Problematic peer functioning in girls with ADHD: A systematic literature review. *PLoS One,* 2016; 11(11):e0165119.

Kooij, J.J., Michielsen, M., Kruithof, H. *et al.* ADHD in old age: A review of the literature and proposal for assessment and treatment. *Expert Review of Neurotherapeutics,* 2016; 16(12):1371–1381.

Kopp, S. Girls with Social and/or Attention Impairments. Doctoral thesis. Gothenburg University, Sweden, 2010.

Kopp, S. & Gillberg, C. Swedish child and adolescent psychiatric out-patients – a five-year cohort. *European Child & Adolescent Psychiatry,* 2003; 12(1):30–35.

Kopp, S., Kelly, K.B. & Gillberg, C. Girls with social and/or attention deficits: A descriptive study of 100 clinic attenders. *Journal of Attention Disorders,* 2010; 14(2):167–181.

Kuja-Halkola, R., Lind Juto, K., Skoglund, C. *et al.* Do borderline personality disorder and attention-deficit/hyperactivity disorder co-aggregate in families? A population-based study of 2 million Swedes. *Molecular Psychiatry,* 2021; 26(1):341–349.

Kuppers, E., Ivanova, T., Karolczak, M. *et al.* Estrogen: A multifunctional messenger to nigrostriatal dopaminergic neurons. *Journal of Neurocytology,* 2000; 29(5–6):375–385.

Kurz, S., Schoebi, D., Dremmel, D. *et al.* Satiety regulation in children with loss of control eating and attention-deficit/hyperactivity disorder: A test meal study. *Appetite,* 2017; 116:90–98.

Larsson, H., Anckarsater, H., Rastam, M., Chang, Z. & Lichtenstein, P. Childhood attention-deficit hyperactivity disorder as an extreme of a continuous trait: A quantitative genetic study of 8,500 twin pairs. *Journal of Child Psychology and Psychiatry,* 2012; 53: 73–80.

Larsson, H., Asherson, P., Chang, Z., Ljung, T. *et al.* Genetic and environmental influences on adult attention deficit hyperactivity disorder symptoms: A large Swedish population based study of twins. *Psychological Medicine,* 2013; 43:197–207.

Leahy, L.G. Attention-Deficit/Hyperactivity Disorder: A Historical Review (1775 to Present). *Journal of Psychosocial Nursing and Mental Health Services.* 2017, 1;55(9):10-16.

Lundin, C., Wikman, A., Wikman, P. *et al*. Hormonal contraceptive use and risk of depression among young women with attention deficit hyperactivity disorder. *Journal of the American Academy of Child and Adolescent Psychiatry*, 2023; 62(6):665–674.

Marangoni, C., De Chiara, L. & Faedda, G.L. Bipolar disorder and ADHD: Comorbidity and diagnostic distinctions. *Current Psychiatry Reports*, 2015; 17(8):604.

Matthies, S.D. & Philipsen, A. Common ground in Attention Deficit Hyperactivity Disorder (ADHD) and Borderline Personality Disorder (BPD): Review of recent findings. *Borderline Personality Disorder Emotional Dysregulation*, 2014; 1:3.

McAllister-Williams, R.H., Baldwin, D.S., Cantwell, R. *et al*. British Association for Psychopharmacology consensus guidance on the use of psychotropic medication preconception, in pregnancy and postpartum 2017. *Journal of Psychopharmacology*, 2017; 31(5):519–552.

Milioni, A.L., Chaim, T.M., Cavallet, M. *et al*. High IQ may 'mask' the diagnosis of ADHD by compensating for deficits in executive functions in treatment-naïve adults with ADHD. *Journal of Attention Disorders*, 2017; 21(6): 455–464.

Miquel, M., Nicola, S.M., Gil-Miravet, I., Guarque-Chabrera, J. & Sanchez-Hernandez, A. A working hypothesis for the role of the cerebellum in impulsivity and compulsivity. *Frontiers in Behavioral Neuroscience*, 2019;13:99.

Mischel, W., Ebbesen, E.B. & Zeiss, A.R. Cognitive and attentional mechanisms in delay of gratification. *Journal of Personality and Social Psychology*, 1972; 21(2):204–218.

Mischel, W., Shoda, Y. & Rodriguez, M.I. Delay of gratification in children. *Science*, 1989; 244(4907):933–938.

Mowlem, F., Agnew-Blais, J., Taylor, E. *et al*. Do different factors influence whether girls versus boys meet ADHD diagnostic criteria? Sex differences among children with high ADHD symptoms. *Psychiatry Research*, 2019a; (272):765–773.

Mowlem, F.D., Rosenqvist, M.A., Martin, J. *et al*. Sex differences in predicting ADHD clinical diagnosis and pharmacological treatment. *European Child & Adolescent Psychiatry*, 2019b; 28:481–489.

Nadeau, K.G.Q.P. *Understanding Women with ADHD*. 2002. Silver Spring, MD: Advantage Books.

Nazar, B.P., de Sousa Pinna, C.M., Suwwan, R. *et al*. ADHD rate in obese women with binge eating and bulimic behaviors from a weight-loss clinic. *Journal of Attention Disorders*, 2016; 20(7):610–616.

Nazar, B.P., Pinna, C.M., Coutinho, G. et al. Review of literature of attention deficit/hyperactivity disorder with comorbid eating disorders. *Brazilian Journal of Psychiatry*, 2008; 30(4):384–389.

Nigg, J.T. Attention-deficit/hyperactivity disorder and adverse health outcomes. *Clinical Psychology Review*, 2013; 33(2):215–228.

Nilsson, I. & Nilsson-Lundmark, E. ADHD ur ett socioekonomiskt perspektiv. *Socialmedicinsk tidskrift*, 2013 (in Swedish).

Ohan, J.L. & Visser, T.A. Why is there a gender gap in children presenting for attention deficit/hyperactivity disorder services? *Journal of Clinical Child and Adolescent Psychology*: the official journal for the Society of Clinical Child and Adolescent Psychology, American Psychological Association, Division 5, 2009; 38(5):650–660.

Østergaard, S.D., Dalsgaard, S., Faraone S.V. et al. Teenage parenthood and birth rates for individuals with and without attention-deficit/hyperactivity disorder: A nationwide cohort study. *Journal of the American Academy of Child & Adolescent Psychiatry*, 2017; 56(7):578–584.

Petrovic, P. *Känslostormar*. Natur & Kultur. 2015 (in Swedish).

Pisecco, S., Huzinec, C. & Curtis, D. The effect of child characteristics on teachers' acceptability of classroom-based behavioral strategies and psychostimulant medication for the treatment of ADHD. *Journal of Clinical Child Psychology*, 2001; 30:413–421.

Polanczyk, G.V., Willcutt, E.G., Salum, G.A. et al. ADHD prevalence estimates across three decades: An updated systematic review and meta-regression analysis. *International Journal of Epidemiology*, 2014; 43(2):434–442.

Quinn, P.O. Treating adolescent girls and women with ADHD: Gender-specific issues. *Journal of Clinical Psychology*, 2005; 61(5):579–587.

Quinn, P.O. & Madhoo, M. A review of attention-deficit/hyperactivity disorder in women and girls: Uncovering this hidden diagnosis. *The Primary Care Companion for CNS Disorders*, 2014; 16(3):PCC.13r01596

Quinn, P.O. & Wigal, S. Perceptions of girls and ADHD: Results from a national survey. *Medscape General Medicine*, 2004; 6(2):2.

van Rensburg, K. & Arif, M. The language of ADHD and its relevance in the diagnostic process. 7th World Congress on ADHD, Lisbon – 25 April 2019.

Roberts, B., Eisenlohr-Moul, T. & Martel, M.M. Reproductive steroids and ADHD symptoms across the menstrual cycle. *Psychoneuroendocrinology*, 2018; 88:105–114.

Rucklidge, J., Brown, D., Crawford, S. et al. Attributional styles and psychosocial functioning of adults with ADHD: Practice issues and gender differences. *Journal of Attention Disorders*, 2007; 10(3):288–298.

Rucklidge, J. & Tannock, R. Psychiatric, psychosocial, and cognitive functioning of female adolescents with ADHD. *Journal of the American Academy of Child and Adolescent Psychiatry*, 2001; 40(5):530–540.

Sanchez, M., Lavigne, R., Romero, J.F. *et al.* Emotion regulation in participants diagnosed with attention deficit hyperactivity disorder, before and after an emotion regulation intervention. *Frontiers in Psychology*, 2019; 10:1092.

SBU. *ADHD hos flickor, en inventering av det vetenskapliga underlaget.* Rapport nr 174, 2005 (in Swedish).

Sciutto, M.J., Nolfi, C.J. & Bluhm, C. Effects of child gender and symptom type on referrals for ADHD by elementary school teachers. *Journal of Emotional and Behavioral Disorders*, 2004; 12:247–253.

SFBUP. *Riktlinje ADHD* www.sfbup.se/vardprogram/riktlinje-adhd (in Swedish).

Skoglund, C., Chen, Q., D'Onofrio, B.M. *et al.* Familial confounding of the association between maternal smoking during pregnancy and ADHD in offspring. *Journal of Child Psychology and Psychiatry*, 2014; 55 61–68

Skoglund, C., Chen, Q., Franck, J. *et al.* Attention-Deficit/Hyperactivity Disorder and risk for substance use disorders in relatives. *Biological Psychiatry*, 2015; 77:880–886

Skoglund, C., Kopp Kallner, H., Skalkidou, A. *et al.* Association of Attention-Deficit/Hyperactivity Disorder with teenage birth among women and girls in Sweden. *JAMA Network Open*, 2019; 2(10):e1912463.

Sonuga-Barke, E.J. & Castellanos, F.X. Spontaneous attentional fluctuations in impaired states and pathological conditions: A neurobiological hypothesis. *Neuroscience & Biobehavioral Review*, 2007; 31(7):977–986.

Sundström Poromaa, I., Comasco, E., Sumner, R. *et al.* Progesterone – friend or foe? *Frontiers in Neuroendocrinology*, 2020; 59:100856.

Surman, C.B.H. & Goodman, D.W. Is ADHD a valid diagnosis in older adults? *Attention Deficit Hyperactivity Disorder,* 2017; 9(3):161–168.

Thapar, A. & Cooper, M. Attention deficit hyperactivity disorder. *The Lancet,* 2016; 387(10024):1240–1250.

Thapar, A., Cooper, M., Eyre, O. *et al.* What have we learnt about the causes of ADHD? *Journal of Child Psychology and Psychiatry, and Allied Disciplines,* 2013; 54(1):3–16.

Thurber, J.R., Heller, T.L. & Hinshaw, S.P. The social behaviors and peer expectation of girls with attention deficit hyperactivity disorder and comparison girls. *Journal of Clinical Child and Adolescent Psychology,* 2002; 31(4):443–452.

University of Chicago. WISER – The Scientific Roots of Wisdom, Compassion, & What Makes us Good. A Discussion with Dilip Jeste and Howard Nusbaum, November 19, 2020.

Weber, M.T., Maki, P.M. & McDermott, M.P. Cognition and mood in perimenopause: A systematic review and meta-analysis. *The Journal of Steroid Biochemistry and Molecular Biology*, 2013; 142:90–98.

White, T.L., Justice, A.J., de Wit, H. Differential subjective effects of D-amphetamine by gender, hormone levels and menstrual cycle phase. *Pharmacology, Biochemistry, and Behavior*, 2002; 73(4):729–741.

Wynchank, D., Bijlenga, D., Beekman, A.T. *et al.* Adult Attention-Deficit/ Hyperactivity Disorder (ADHD) and insomnia: An update of the literature. *Current Psychiatry Reports*, 2017; 19(12):98.

Wynchank, D., Ten Have, M., Bijlenga, D. *et al.* The association between insomnia and sleep duration in adults with Attention-Deficit Hyperactivity Disorder: Results from a general population study. *Journal of Clinical Sleep Medicine*: official publication of the American Academy of Sleep Medicine, 2018; 14(3):349–357.

Young, S., Adamo, N., Ásgeirsdóttir, B.B. *et al.* Females with ADHD: An expert consensus statement taking a lifespan approach providing guidance for the identification and treatment of attention-deficit/ hyperactivity disorder in girls and women. *BMC Psychiatry*, 2020; 20(1):404.